DO-IT-YOURSELF MEDICAL TESTING

DO-IT-YOURSELF MEDICAL TESTING

MORE THAN 160 TESTS YOU CAN DO AT HOME

Cathey Pinckney

and

Edward R. Pinckney, M.D.

Illustrations by the Authors

Medical examinations and observations you can perform on yourself and your family to help you participate actively in your health care, prevent certain diseases, monitor some illnesses and maintain good health

(1983)

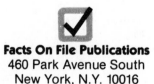

Facts On File Publications
460 Park Avenue South
New York, N.Y. 10016

FOR C.L.P.

Great Librarian, Great Shooter, but still a **Bum***

*(From Neil Simon's "Come Blow Your Horn")

Do It Yourself Medical Tests

Library of Congress Cataloging in Publication Data

Pinckney, Cathey.
  Do-it-yourself medical testing.

  Includes indexes.
  1. Diagnosis. 2. Self-examination, Medical.
I. Pinckney, Edward R. II. Title.
RC71.3.P56 1981   616.07'5   82-12069
ISBN 0-87196-705-7

Printed and bound in the United States of America

9 8 7 6 5 4 3 2

PLEASE NOTE

Should you have any problem with a medical test device or supplies, after assuring yourself that the test was performed properly, you can help yourself and others by reporting that problem to:

Medical Device & Laboratory Product Problem Reporting Program*

Call toll free anytime: 800–638–6725

Problems that have already been reported, and in most instances corrected, include:

* Directions not clear, inadequate or seem to be wrong
* The test was difficult to perform
* The device or test material does not seem to perform properly
* The device or test material does not seem safe to handle or operate
* The device, or parts of it, break easily
* The test results do not seem appropriate or consistent, especially after checking with your doctor's office or a commercial laboratory
* The container or bottle as part of a test kit can easily be mistaken for some other medicinal product
* The product was labelled wrong.

* A cooperative venture of the United States Pharmacopeia, the federal Food and Drug Administration and the American College of Physicians

CONTENTS

INTRODUCTION

There is nothing new about home medical testing. If you have ever taken your own or your child's temperature, or simply felt for the warmth of a forehead, you have performed no less of a medical test than your doctor does when he or she takes your blood pressure or taps your knee with a rubber reflex hammer—both of which you can also do. You can just as easily measure how much glucose (sugar) is in your blood and urine, examine your feces for hidden blood and worms, evaluate your vision and hearing, and even appraise how well your heart and lungs are functioning. In fact, there are more than 160 medical tests that can be performed at home.

In most instances the cost of home testing will be far less than the cost of testing carried out in a doctor's office, hospital or commercial laboratory. But of even greater importance, the test results can be far more accurate. When you realize that about one in every seven professionally performed medical tests is either in error or unreliable for practical application, that little bit of extra care and attention you provide when you test yourself can make quite a difference as far as accuracy is concerned. Furthermore, blood pressure observations are far more accurate when measured in familiar surroundings, and blood glucose values are much more precise and useful when they reflect your typical daily activities rather than the apprehension you feel in your doctor's office or the effects you experience after lying in a hospital bed for several days.

WHAT MEDICAL TESTS DO

Most people think medical tests make diagnoses. The tests alone do not. They are rarely specific about any disease. Tests do *help* confirm the cause of an illness, usually by pointing toward one condition more than others that can cause similar symptoms. They may aid in locating the source of pain or discomfort. They can, at times, assist in relieving the anguish that accompanies so many medical conditions. (It is a known fact that many people feel completely cured of their complaints without any therapy whatsoever simply after undergoing one or more tests.) But in all but a very few instances, tests are not precise.

The detection of hidden (also called occult) blood in your bowel movement, for instance, does not necessarily mean disease—least of all colon cancer. The occult blood test (occult means not visible to the naked eye) can be positive for several days after you eat rare meat; after you brush your teeth, especially if you brush your gums properly; after you take aspirin, vitamin C or iron tablets. Or occult blood could come from parasites acquired simply by going barefoot; dogs can deposit worms in backyards or on lawns, and these worms can bore through the skin and settle in the intestines.

The fact that most medical tests are ambiguous is only one drawback. Their accuracy and usefulness are further compromised by a variety of bodily aberrations, routine activities and environmental conditions. Whether you sit or stand when you take a test can alter the resulting value, as can what you eat or drink. A loud noise or a pretty nurse can so distort a blood cholesterol test's outcome as to result in unnecessary diet and other life-style changes. In other words, do not rely on medical tests alone. If they corroborate your medical history (your description of your illness, including your past health record and that of your family, is probably the most important of all clues that ultimately lead to a diagnosis), and if the tests parallel the direction of your signs and symptoms (signs are objective indicators, such as a rash; symptoms are subjective, such as pain), then the tests become just another link in the chain that should support a correct clinical conclusion followed by successful specific therapy.

HEALTH MAINTENANCE

Where home medical testing can be of real value is in screening for early warning signs of some inconspicuous or latent diseases—especially when timely detection can prevent disability. Home testing can be of equal value when used to monitor and help control some existing illnesses. When people with diabetes were taught to test their own blood glucose levels at home, the dangerous consequences of diabetic coma were reduced by almost 70 percent, and the number of emergency visits to doctors and hospitals was halved. In another self-care program for patients with an inherited blood disease, the cost of medical care was reduced by over half, and the life span of these patients was more than doubled.

Many medical tests consist of nothing more than observation: the secret simply lies in knowing what to watch for and what the perceived information could mean. If all parents would kiss the cheeks and foreheads of their infants regularly and learn to discern any unusual saltiness on the skin surface, many of the tragic lung and intestinal problems that can result from cystic fibrosis could probably be prevented. If family members would learn to observe each other's ears, eyes, throats and skin, they could at times become aware of medical versus nonmedical conditions and relieve themselves of much anxiety—not to mention expense. Simple systematic scrutiny of one's breasts, hair, feces, teeth, temperature, testicles, urine and weight are home medical tests that can repay the effort a thousandfold in physical and financial peace of mind. Knowing what questions to ask an elderly family member who is behaving in a seemingly abnormal manner could help differentiate between a physical or psychological basis for the problem. Using the right questionnaire has been known to prevent tragic social and financial consequences in many a family where incipient brain and liver abnormalities had been overlooked.

If home medical testing does nothing more than prompt you to seek medical care early enough to allow a simple, relatively comfortable cure, it is more than justified. And lest you think that the medical profession discourages this seeming intrusion into its hallowed halls, direct participation in one's own health care, as well as in the care of family members, is now accepted within the medical profession. Most doctors encourage their patients to play a part in arriving at a diagnosis and welcome shared responsibility in making treatment choices. They have found that this not only increases patient compliance, allowing a more rapid, more successful outcome, but it is also an effective means of preventing related health problems.

SOME PRECAUTIONS

While most of the medical tests described in this book are fairly easy to perform, and the equipment or supplies needed are relatively inexpensive, they should not be thought of as playthings. Directions that accompany test material should be followed exactly. It is recommended that the first time any test is performed, it be done in consultation with your doctor. Let him or her watch you take your blood pressure initially; let your physician show you how to take your own blood sample; let him or her demonstrate visual field testing, the use of the reflex hammer, tuning fork, otoscope and any other instrument you contemplate using. In this way, you can avoid many misunderstandings and errors.

Practice using your instruments at home on family and friends you know are in good health. Look at normal eardrums or throats; observe the effect of reflex testing; observe urine consistency, body blemishes and contours as often as possible. The more familiar you become with such things, the more accurate your test results.

Because so many of the tests depend on color comparisons, be sure you have normal color vision as well as good visual acuity. Do not attempt to evaluate color changes if you have any doubt about your ability to discriminate between colors.

Always keep in mind, too, the possibility of false-positive and false-negative results. A false-positive test is one that indicates the possible presence of the disease or condition when that disease or condition does not exist. The more sensitive a test is, the more likely that a false-positive result can occur. Diet, physical activity, emotional upset, the medicines you take and failure to follow test directions exactly are also apt to alter or falsify a test's results. A false-negative test is one that fails to show a positive result even though some disease or condition exists that should cause a positive value. More often than not, a false-negative result comes from carelessness in performing a test.

Most doctors insist on any medical test being performed twice before incorporating the result into their record of related evidence. Unless performing a home test while under a doctor's care (such as with asthma, diabetes, stomach ulcers or during pregnancy), it is considered good practice to repeat home medical tests at least twice, until you feel sufficiently self-assured about your technique.

MEDICAL CONSULTATION VERSUS MEDICAL ATTENTION

Considering that most home testing will be of the screening or health-monitoring variety, the chances of true positive test results are slim. But should a medical test and its repeat show a positive result suggesting some disease or condition, professional confirmation should be sought. Most positive tests do not indicate an emergency (there are exceptions if you are diabetic, pregnant, etc.) and only warrant a *medical consultation*. That could mean nothing more than a phone conversation with your doctor describing your findings and having the doctor weigh your test results in light of his or her knowledge of your past medical history and his or her last examination of you. It could also mean an office visit to allow additional procedures to confirm or disprove your test findings.

A medical test result that warrants *medical attention* is not necessarily diagnostic, but it could indicate the possibility of some serious or even life-threatening condition as well as a disease that could be dangerous to others around you. If the description of a test in this book advises that medical attention is warranted based on certain test results, this means you should seek immediate medical care, either from your own doctor or—should your personal physician not be available—from a hospital or community emergency facility.

SELF-CARE

Self-care does not necessarily mean assuming total and absolute responsibility for your health; it really means taking a greater interest in, and sharing responsibility for, maintaining good health and participating in diagnosis and therapy. The more you know and understand about disease, the greater your opportunity to apply appropriate measures to avoid illness. Gone is the era when doctors played God, and no one should tolerate a physician who refuses to explain how a sickness came about, how it affects the body and mind, how treatment is supposed to work and all the risks and alternatives involved. Home medical test monitoring is part of preventive maintenance for your body. Remember, no single medical test, whether performed at home, in your doctor's office, in a hospital, or at a commercial laboratory or other test location (X-ray facility, health fair, research center) should be considered diagnostic. This book is not about self-care, as such, but rather provides health information on only one small aspect of health maintenance. It is not a handbook for self-diagnosis but only a guide to help you and your doctor help yourself. A medical test in itself is relatively meaningless until it is interpreted in light of your medical history, your signs and symptoms, and your doctor's training and experience applied to his or her observations after examining you.

WARNINGS

If you have any gross abnormality (pains or persistent aches, growths on your skin, obvious blood in a bowel movement or unexplained bleeding anywhere, difficulty in breathing, inability to coordinate your movements, problems in seeing or hearing, or any discomfort or disability that is more than you have had or are used to), do not rely on any home test before seeking medical attention; call or visit your doctor or emergency center immediately.

Never assume that the result of your medical test is definitive; if you have any doubt about either a positive or a negative test result, consult your physician and share your doubts as well as your test results with him or her.

Every medical test includes some degree of risk; in most instances it is virtually negligible, but every test should be considered from the standpoint of the possible harm it might cause as well as the information it might provide.

• One risk is the possibility that additional, more dangerous tests could be performed in order to substantiate your test findings. Before undergoing sophisticated testing, have your doctor assure you of its necessity; that there are no alternative, safer tests; and that the results of the tests will affect or alter your doctor's decisions.
• The other, equally serious risk is that a false-negative test result can offer misleading assurance that you are disease-free; never make that absolute assumption without your doctor's confirmation.

And this is not a book on home treatment. No suggestions, recommendations or directions are meant to be offered as therapy or any other means to a cure. True, a good scrubbing in a hot tub might help eliminate fleas, lice or mites, but the real remedy for any condition comes from working with your doctor to assure the success of treatment and the avoidance of possible complications. Let home medical testing be your means of maintaining your health and preventing disease; but let it be no more than your adjunct to professional diagnosis and treatment.

HOW TO USE THIS BOOK

The tests presented in this book are grouped under various categories not necessarily related to the conditions their results can reflect. Urine tests, for example, can indicate a wide variety of bodily actions or reactions not limited to the kidneys and genitourinary system. Blood tests can suggest problems outside the circulatory system. A breath test for alcohol really has no bearing on how well the lungs function. The simplest way to decide on a test is to first ascertain its purpose. If a medical test is intended to screen for the possibility of latent disease, the "Health Maintenance Index" (Appendix I) should be consulted. Should the possibility of some specific condition be in mind, refer to the "Disease-Related Index" (Appendix II). When your doctor recommends a particular test, the Table of Contents should suffice.

The introduction to each test describes its general purpose, what substance or function it is supposed to indicate or measure, how the test works and any common conditions (activities, diet, drugs, etc.) that could interfere with the test results. This preliminary discussion is not intended to be all-inclusive; it is nothing more than a basic, simply worded explanation of what the test is about.

Each test description includes the sections discussed below.

What Is Usual
Because it is almost impossible to define "normal" values without due regard for a particular individual's age, sex, height, weight, family characteristics and a host of other variables, this section describes what one would most likely find in the "average" person. Should routine activities tend to alter test values in a supposedly healthy human being, the effect of such activities is mentioned. For example, physical exercise or prolonged walking or standing can cause a positive urine protein test, but it could be a normal, rather than abnormal, test result for many people. And many test results are not simply positive or negative; some show quantitative changes, such as when measuring how much air the lungs can hold. In almost all medical tests, *usual* values can fluctuate widely and still be usual.

What You Need
Personal abilities as well as required equipment and/or supplies are listed, along with approximate costs. For some tests the price for the material will

seem high, either because the manufacturer packages the material only in large quantities at this time, or because the necessary apparatus is costly. To offset the cost of expensive items, many people form groups or use clubs or other organizations to share the cost and use of such paraphernalia. Others weigh the cost against travel time and expenditures for repeated visits to the doctor's office when the same test can be performed at home; for example, a spirometer to monitor asthma and other chest ailments can pay for itself just by eliminating the need for two office visits.

The cost of equipment or supplies can vary tremendously from one pharmacy or medical supply store to the next. There are no fixed prices for test material, so it can pay to shop around. The prices cited in this book were typical at the time of publication.

In a great many instances, health insurance plans or government-sponsored medical care programs will reimburse you, in part or fully, for the purchase of a medical device or test material when recommended by a physician. "At-home" blood glucose monitors and blood pressure measuring machines are only two examples of medical equipment usually covered by insurance reimbursement for rental or purchase.

The easiest place to find most of the items needed for testing is your local pharmacy. While not every item will always be carried in stock, pharmacists have access to wholesale medical supply houses. Check the Yellow Pages of your telephone directory under the headings "Hospital Equipment & Supplies" and "Physicians' and Surgeons' Equipment & Supplies" for sources of supplies unavailable at or through your pharmacy. Many of these home health care businesses also rent expensive test apparatus. Abbey Medical and Bard Home Health franchises are but two examples of nationwide dealers; they offer comprehensive catalogs without charge. Sears Roebuck has a free home health catalog, and some direct-mail catalogs, such as those from Hammacher Schlemmer in New York City or The Sharper Image in San Francisco, include medical test devices. If you have a good relationship with your doctor, he or she can easily order anything and everything you could need from a pharmaceutical supply house at the lowest possible cost.

At times you may be confronted by a pharmacist or medical supply sales representative who will refuse to sell you a test item unless you present a doctor's prescription. With very few exceptions, the test material described in this book does not, by law, require a doctor's permission for purchase. Where such devices are so restricted, however, most doctors usually supply the device directly. As one example, the GONODECTEN test kit (see **Genitourinary System** tests, **Gonorrhea** test) is often given to the patient to perform at home. If the doctor is not aware of the test result, he or she is not obligated to report the individual and the disease to public health authorities—as the law requires the doctor to do should he or she become aware of the condition. (Another home gonorrhea test, VD ALERT, needs no prescription.) You can always contact your local FDA office to determine the status of any specific device.

As a convenience, manufacturers of commonly used equipment and supplies are listed in the Appendix III section at the end of the book.

What to Watch Out For
The majority of the caveats mentioned in this section reflect the mistakes and problems people have experienced when performing a particular test. They are primarily observations of mechanical difficulties to be avoided, but they also include commonly overlooked possible interferences with proper test procedures as well as technical obstacles that may arise.

Although the products and supplies mentioned in this book were available at the time of publication, it is possible that technological developments might well cause a device or test material to be withdrawn from the marketplace or be replaced by something different—usually something easier to use and more effective. The home diagnostics field is growing so rapidly that it is difficult to keep track of every new device. The federal Food and Drug Administration (FDA) Bureau of Medical Devices, which evaluates every piece of medical equipment before it is allowed to be sold—from thermometers to pregnancy test kits and even wooden tongue depressors—has reviewed 17,500 notices of intent to market a medical device since 1976, when the Medical Device Amendments law was passed, and still has a backlog of 44,800 products under study. On the average it recalls about 150 devices annually. Should you have any question about the efficacy or safety of any test equipment, contact your local FDA office.

However, you should watch out for expiration dates on supplies that require them. Be sure that the material you buy will have a reasonable shelf life. And be sure the product is properly sealed; many chemicals become useless when exposed to air or moisture.

What the Test Results Can Mean
The conditions described in this section are suggestive of the most common causes of abnormal or unusual test results. You should never attempt to interpret a "positive" or abnormal test result yourself. As but one example, a lower-than-normal blood hemoglobin test, while most likely signifying an anemia, does not even hint at what is causing the anemia. Medical textbooks list anemia as part of, or the consequence of, several hundred unrelated diseases. Then again, the test result could have come from your squeezing your fingertip too tightly and diluting the drop of blood with other tissue fluids.

Although any one of the implications noted here may seem quite plausible, it would be a foolish waste of time and testing to accept such test results as conclusive. Should a test result warrant a medical consultation, it would be a disservice to yourself and your family not to contact your doctor and discuss the matter. Should a test result warrant medical attention, it would be irresponsible not to proceed immediately to your doctor or nearest emergency facility.

If, however, your test results do not indicate ill health, and you take pleasure in monitoring and maintaining your health as well as preventing illness, enjoy!

URINE TESTS

Urinalysis probably offers more health information with less effort and at less cost than any other medical test procedure. The examination and evaluation of urine and its contents can reveal a wealth of knowledge about the human body, including:

- Urinary tract disorders—kidney, bladder, prostate and urethral disease as well as related nerve and nutritional problems that affect the urinary tract
- Abuses to the body—poisoning or drug use
- Blood production and utilization
- The possibility of cancer
- Genetic or inherited conditions
- Hormone activity
- Infections outside the urinary system
- Liver and gallbladder functioning
- Metabolism of carbohydrates, fats and proteins
- Nutritional status—including vitamin and mineral utilization
- Parasitic invasion
- Pulmonary (lung) functioning.

In addition, regular self-testing of urine can be invaluable in maintaining one's health, providing early warning signs of impending illness, keeping track of an existing disease to avoid complications and evaluating the efficacy of therapy.

Urine is a solution of end products of almost all the various metabolic cell functions in the body. These waste products are carried by the blood to the kidneys, from which they are excreted as urine, which also includes excess fluids and the minerals that help control water excretion and retention.

There are at least 20 different tests that can be performed at home on a urine sample—technically called a urine specimen. More than half of these tests require nothing more than inserting a dipstick (a chemically treated strip of thin plastic) into the urine and then comparing it to a standard color chart

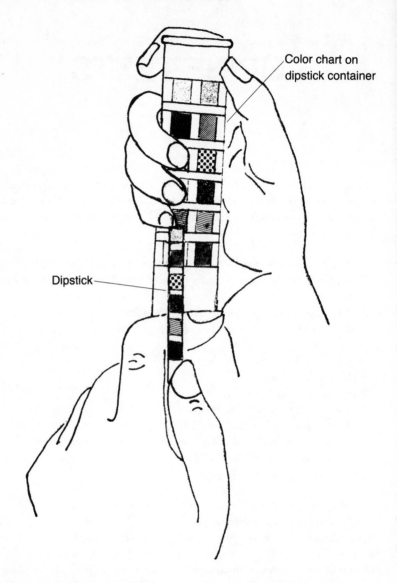

Color chart on dipstick container

Dipstick

Figure 1. Dipstick urine testing (six different test measurements).

on the side of the dipstick container (Figure 1). Four of the remaining tests require nothing more than careful observations, and the rest require only a simple, inexpensive apparatus.

Always keep in mind that if you are taking any medicine or vitamins or have eaten any unusual foods (e.g., beets) prior to performing a urine test, these things can interfere with test results. For example, if you regularly take vitamin C, it can cause a false-negative reaction in a test for infection; that is, even when an infection is present, excessive vitamin C in the urine will make the test results suggest that no infection exists. The most common foods, drugs and other body activities that can alter test results are noted in the description of each test. Do not hesitate to check with your doctor or pharmacist to ascertain the specific name of each drug you are taking.

OBTAINING A URINE SAMPLE

What You Need
- A clean, dry, container, preferably made of clear glass, with a capacity of at least 16 ounces (one pint); the opening or mouth of the container should be wide enough to allow urination into the container without difficulty; if urine is to be tested for a possible infection, the receptacle should first be placed in a pan, covered with water and boiled for 20 minutes, then drained and carefully air-dried; the inside surfaces should not be touched; an easy-to-use, inexpensive, reusable urine-collection device is described in the **Urine Flow Rate** test
- Sterile gauze or cotton, especially when you are testing for an infection
- A dipstick testing device; the specific kind required is described in the entry on each test; while some dipsticks measure only a single urine component or condition, there are others that perform 10 different tests at one time; these multiple-test strips are best for general urine screening; one brand is the N-Multistix SG, which costs from $30.00 to $35.00 for a package of 100 test strips; another is the Chemstrip 9, at a similar cost
- Chek-Stix—these are control sticks that will allow you to determine whether your dipsticks are in good condition and whether you are performing the test properly; they are optional and cost $17.00 for a package of 25.

Dipstick testing is considered as accurate as intricate chemical analysis in almost all the evaluations it can perform; many hospitals and physicians' laboratories use dipstick testing routinely, sending urine specimens for chemical evaluation only as required to confirm unusual abnormal results.

The Clean-Catch Specimen
For certain urine tests, especially those designed to detect the presence of blood or to indicate the presence of an infection, a clean-catch specimen is preferred to avoid any possible contamination. Here is how to obtain such a specimen:

- An uncircumcised man should pull back the foreskin of the penis and

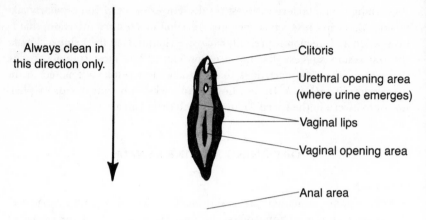

Figure 2. Female genital area.

wipe the tip with warm, soapy water and then rinse before collecting the specimen

- A woman should spread the lips of the vaginal opening and wash the area surrounding the urethral opening with warm, soapy water and rinse; the urine should be passed while the vaginal lips are held apart (Figure 2); this is especially important during menstruation or if there is a vaginal discharge; when washing or wiping the urethral opening area, be sure to wipe only from front to back, never from back to front, to avoid any contamination from the anal area

- A midvoid specimen is preferred, if at all possible; this means that the first and last portions of urine should not be allowed to enter the urine container; the exception to this rule is the **Two/Three-Glass** test

   (Note: a T-Tube Clean Catch System containing all necessary supplies and instructions is available from Whale Scientific, Inc., 4945 Monaco, Commerce City, CO 80022 at $1.25 per kit with a minimum order of three)

- While urine passed at any time of the day is usually satisfactory for testing, the best specimen is the one passed immediately after awakening in the morning.

What to Watch Out For

- If blood seems to be visible in the urine, home testing should be avoided and medical attention sought immediately
- Dipsticks must be kept in a tightly closed container and in a cool, dry place away from light and heat
- If in doubt about the quality of a dipstick, verify its accuracy by utilizing a Chek-Stix; you can also compare the dipstick's various colors to the test charts when dry and then dip the dipstick in distilled water to note any

color change; there should be none; many doctors believe that dipsticks should not be used more than four months after the time the bottle containing them was opened, regardless of the expiration date printed on the container

• Because urine components are evaluated with dipsticks through color comparisons, do not attempt such test interpretations if you have any color vision impairment; have someone with normal color vision "read" your test results.

BILIRUBIN

Bilirubin is formed from the hemoglobin in red blood cells after they break down at the end of their usual life span (four months). It is a gold-colored pigment that is excreted primarily by the bowel and helps give feces their dark color. Usually, the urine color will range from a very dark yellow to brown if abnormal amounts of bilirubin are present, especially if the urine sample forms a yellow foam when shaken. Many different antibiotics, hormones, tranquilizers, diuretics and pain relievers can cause a positive urine bilirubin test, as can prolonged alcoholism. The yellow color of jaundice seen in the eyes and skin is usually caused by excessive amounts of bilirubin in the blood, and, in fact, the test for bilirubin is most often performed when some form of liver disease is suspected, since a positive urine test can occur before the rest of the body reflects liver damage. While the test can also reflect some forms of anemia, when this is suspected, the urine **Urobilinogen** test should also be performed.

What Is Usual
Not even a trace of bilirubin should be detected in the urine.

What You Need
Any one of several different dipstick testing strips: Most Chemstrips and Multistix incorporate this test and cost approximately $20.00 to $25.00 for 100 test strips.

What to Watch Out For
The urine must be fresh and kept from prolonged exposure to light. Because so many drugs can interfere with the test, check with your doctor or pharmacist to ascertain if a medicine you are taking will affect the test. A urinary infection can cause a false-negative test (see Urine Tests, **Leukocyte** and **Nitrite** tests). The test strips must be fresh, and because the color change is so slight, excellent color vision is essential.

What the Test Results Can Mean
Any indication of bilirubin in the urine warrants a medical consultation. If there are other symptoms (fever, jaundice, lethargy), medical attention should be sought. A positive test can be an early warning signal of hepatitis, and immediate medical attention can help ward off cirrhosis of the liver. Some other conditions, such as gallstones, cancer and even thyroid disease, may be signaled by a positive urine bilirubin test. And although drug use may cause a positive test, the test could also reflect liver damage from drugs or alcohol.

BLOOD

If obvious blood is seen in urine, especially in a midvoid specimen, immediate medical attention should be sought. In most instances, however, when blood is present in urine, it is "occult" (present, but not visible). The test detects hemoglobin and red blood cells. When performed along with the urine **Two/ Three-Glass** test, it is sometimes possible to locate the source of the occult blood. Many drugs, such as pain relievers, certain tranquilizers, some antihistamine products, anticoagulants and a few antibiotics (especially the sulfas), irritate the kidneys to a point where occult blood will be found in the urine. In rare instances, excessive exertion or exercise causes occult blood in urine, but this is not considered a disease. Obviously, menstruation can cause a false-positive urine blood test.

What Is Usual
No indication of blood should be detected in urine; even if there seems to be a logical explanation for a positive test, such as exercise, a positive test warrants medical attention.

What You Need
One of the dipstick-type tests is easiest to use and is sufficiently accurate for home testing. The Hemastix strips will test for blood alone and cost approximately $4.00 for 50 strips. Most other multiple-test strips include testing for blood in the urine and range in price from $13.00 to $27.00 per 100 test strips, depending on the number of different tests included.

What to Watch Out For
If the urine contains large amounts of vitamin C (see Urine Tests, **Vitamin C** test) or has a high **specific gravity**, the test may show a false-negative result and should not be considered accurate. If you have a urinary tract infection, the test may be false-positive. The test strips must be fresh, and good color vision is necessary.

What the Test Results Can Mean
A positive urine blood test warrants medical attention, if only to eliminate any extraneous cause. Various forms of anemia, especially the inherited kinds such as sickle-cell anemia (see Blood Tests, **Sickle Cell** test), and other blood disorders can cause blood in the urine. Many different diseases such as systemic lupus erythematosis and other immunologically caused conditions can initially manifest themselves by a positive urine blood test. A severe burn, electric shock, crushing-type injury, various poisons such as arsenic and even high blood pressure can cause a positive test. Kidney stones may cause occult blood in the urine before they cause pain. Virtually any urinary tract infection, including prostate disease, parasitic infestation, along with many systemic infections such as malaria or pneumonia, can cause a positive test.

COLOR

The color of urine can reflect many different conditions—from illness to drug use (there are more than 100 commonly used drugs that alter urine color). Exposure to industrial chemicals can also be identified by a change in urine color. While it can be something of a shock to notice an abrupt difference in the color of your urine, it can also be an early warning sign of some impending disease. Then again, it can also be nothing more than a consequence of your diet; and it can be quite a relief to learn that your reddish colored urine is not blood but beets.

What Is Usual
Most of the time urine color ranges from light yellow to dark amber; the greater the volume of urine, usually along with a lessened amount of dissolved material (dilution), the more apt it is to be lighter or paler in color (see Urine Tests, **Specific Gravity** test). After strenuous exercise, excessive sweating or a greatly reduced fluid intake, urine usually assumes a darker color.

What You Need
A clear glass container and good color vision.

What to Watch Out For
Do not forget to take into consideration any drug you are taking; check with your doctor or pharmacist to see if your medicine does affect urine color. Menstruating women may show pink or red-colored urine.

What the Test Results Can Mean
Pink to red to brown or brown-black colored urine, without a definite food or drug explanation, should first be considered to contain blood (red blood

cells and hemoglobin). The urine **Blood** test can help verify the presence of blood. If the test for blood is positive, immediate medical attention should be sought. Red-orange, pink or red urine can also be due to:

- Foods such as beets, blackberries and rhubarb
- Food coloring
- Laxatives such as Ex-Lax, Dorbane, Modane and Senekot
- Drugs, especially some tranquilizers such as Thorazine, Mellaril and Haldol—to name but a very few
- Porphyrins; this can mean liver disease, exposure to toxic chemicals or drug abuse, and if no other explanation is obvious, a medical consultation is warranted.

A vivid yellow or yellow-orange color not subsequent to exercise or other explainable cause of concentrated urine can be due to:

- Anemia
- Thyroid disease
- Decreased kidney function
- Foods such as carrots
- Drugs such as the sulfa medications, cascara laxatives and warfarin products.

The chances of kidney disease are such that a repeated yellow-colored urine warrants medical consultation.

Urine color of green to blue-green could result from:

- Liver or gallbladder trouble (see Urine Tests, **Bilirubin** and **Urobilinogen** tests)
- Use of drugs such as Indocin, for treating arthritis and gout; antidepressants such as Elavil.

Black or very dark urine could suggest the presence of melanin (a pigment of skin cancer), or it could reflect old blood that remained in the bladder. Such a finding warrants medical consultation.

And then, if urine seems consistently colorless, especially when accompanied by excessive volume, it could be an early sign of diabetes: (see Urine Tests, **Glucose** and **Volume** tests). Profuse urination warrants medical consultation.

GLUCOSE

Although urine may contain traces of several kinds of sugar (glucose, fructose, galactose, etc.), the usual test for sugar in the urine is the one specifically for glucose (see Blood Tests, **Glucose** test). Normal glucose (carbohydrate) metabolism is such that most people rarely have a positive test for glucose in their urine. If glucose is repeatedly detected in urine, it usually means that the amount of glucose in the blood is elevated—most commonly due to diabetes (but urine glucose levels alone are not to be considered a reliable indicator of blood glucose levels). When blood and urine glucose tests are performed together, they can indicate how high blood glucose levels must go before the kidneys filter the glucose from the blood into the urine.

While urine specimens can be tested at any time of the day, for this particular test most doctors prefer the second morning specimen (after discarding the first one on awakening), since it better reflects blood sugar levels. A first morning specimen tends to be an accumulation of all urine filtered by the kidneys during the night and is therefore less indicative of diet and metabolism.

As with so many tests, there are a number of non-disease-related factors that can cause a positive glucose test, but the test should become negative once the factor, or factors, are eliminated. They include positive results under the following circumstances:

- After eating extremely large amounts of refined sugar or sugar-containing foods
- After extreme physical exertion
- During and immediately after extreme anxiety or emotional upset
- Along with the use of many different drugs: adrenalin and related medicines used to treat allergies, certain digitalis preparations, some aspirin-containing products, most steroid (cortisone–like) drugs, most diuretics, a few forms of penicillin, barbiturates and drug abuse with narcotics such as morphine.

Note: Patients who know they have diabetes should only follow their doctors' advice on urine glucose testing.

What Is Usual
No glucose should be detected in urine (non–disease exceptions have been cited above). It was once believed that it took a blood glucose level of 180 mg per 100 ml or more before blood sugar would pass through the kidneys into the urine and that a combination of an elevated blood glucose level plus a positive urine glucose test automatically meant diabetes. Recent research has

shown, however, that some "normal" people may have blood sugar levels anywhere from 140 to 240 mg per 100 ml before they "spill" sugar into the urine;
several other tests, such as the blood glucose tolerance test, are now required
before a diagnosis of diabetes can be made.

What You Need

A dipstick-type testing strip such as the Chemstrip G, Clinistix or Diastix (many
people find the Diastix is the easiest to read); these test strips limit their findings to glucose determinations and cost from $2.00 to $3.00 for a bottle of 50
strips. TES-TAPE comes as a continuous roll of test paper (much like a Scotch
Tape dispenser) and costs $3.50 for a minimum of 100 tests; many doctors
feel this is the most accurate paper-type test because it is least affected by
drugs. Multiple-test dipsticks usually contain glucose as one of the 9 or 10
tests on the strip and cost from $25.00 to $30.00 for 100 strips.

What to Watch Out For

- Many of these tests depend on time measurements that must be followed
  exactly to avoid false results; the time is not the same for all the tests
- Be sure the test strips are not old and are in good working order (see the
  discussion of Chex-stix in the urine testing introduction)
- Do not attempt color-change interpretation unless you have normal color
  vision
- If you are taking large doses of vitamin C, an excess of this vitamin in
  the urine can cause a false-positive test (see Urine Tests, **Vitamin C** test);
  do not take vitamin C for three days prior to testing for urine glucose
- Antibiotics, aspirin products and vitamin C can cause a false-positive test
  when using Diastix; the same products may cause a false-negative test
  when using Clinistix or TES-TAPE
- Be sure to take into account any medicine you are using (even one you
  bought without a prescription); a recent study showed that one out of
  three inaccurate urine glucose tests were the result of ignoring a drug or
  forgetting to take it into account.

What the Test Results Can Mean

Urine glucose tests that are positive for two or three days in a row warrant
medical consultation, even if there is a possible extraneous cause—if only to
rule out a disease process. In most instances, however, repeated positive glucose reactions indicate diabetes, especially if there is a family history of the
disease. But because a positive urine glucose test could mean some other hormone disorder—faulty glucose metabolism can reflect adrenal, pituitary or
thyroid gland disorders—as well as the latent consequence of an old heart
attack, little strokes, liver disease or even an old brain injury, a diagnosis of

diabetes is not absolute until confirmed by additional testing. Some infectious diseases, such as pancreatitis, may also cause a positive glucose test.

KETONES

Ketones, sometimes called ketone bodies, are composed of two different acids and acetone. They can reflect the metabolism (utilization) of fat and fatty acids in the body. When there are insufficient carbohydrates available to supply energy, the liver usually starts converting fat to energy as an alternative, and this is reflected by the presence of ketones in the urine (a condition called ketonuria). Because people with diabetes have problems with carbohydrate metabolism, they are most apt to show ketones in the urine. There are, however, other circumstances that provoke ketonuria:

- An inadequate food intake, usually over several days, or even severe vomiting can cause the body to produce excess ketones
- A diet that omits virtually all carbohydrates (the Atkin's diet utilizes urine ketone measurements as an indicator of adherence)
- Conditions that interfere with proper digestion
- Diseases that cause a high fever
- The use of certain medicines can cause a false-positive reaction (some drugs used to treat the symptoms of Parkinson's disease and a few sleeping preparations).

This test is primarily one for known diabetics to use as an additional means of following the course of their disease.

What Is Usual
Ketone bodies should not be detected in the urine.

What You Need
Either one of the dipstick test strips specifically for ketones only, such as Chemstrip K or Ketostix, or the Acetest tablet test, which cost approximately $6.00 per 100 strips or tablets. Most other multiple-test strips include ketones as part of the battery; their prices range from $15.00 to $30.00 for 100 test strips.

What to Watch Out For
- Do not test a urine specimen that has been left standing for more than 30 minutes; it can give a false-negative reaction
- The color comparison chart for ketone testing is not easy to read; it is suggested that two people evaluate the color change

• The ketone testing chemicals in the strips may fail to change color if they have been exposed to air even for short periods of time; be sure the test strips are fresh and have been properly stored (this caution is more for patients with diabetes who test for ketones as an advance warning against the possibility of diabetic coma).

One way to check on the effectiveness of ketone testing strips is to put a drop of nail polish remover containing acetone on the test area; the acetone should cause a color change. Many patients with diabetes use the tablet test to be sure of the accuracy of the results; the tablets are also more stable over a period of time.

What the Test Results Can Mean
A positive ketone test in a patient with diabetes is sufficient warning to seek immediate medical attention. A persistent positive ketone test in someone without evident diabetes warrants medical consultation.

LEUKOCYTE

A leukocyte is a white blood cell, of which there are many types. They are particularly important in helping to fight infections, and when there is an infection or inflammation in the body, the amount of leukocytes usually increases at the site of the infection. Thus, any noticeable increase in leukocytes in the urine usually indicates an infection somewhere in the urinary tract (kidneys, ureters, bladder, urethra, plus the prostate in men). The test helps confirm the urine **Nitrite** test as an indication of a urinary tract infection.

What Is Usual
It is normal to find a few leukocytes in urine, and women seem to have more leukocytes than men, but these should never amount to more than a trace when tested by a dipstick color indicator.

What You Need
A dipstick-type test strip such as the Chemstrip L, which costs approximately $10.00 per 100 strips. The Chemstrip 9 dipstick performs the leukocyte test and nine additional urine tests, including urine **Nitrite**, and costs approximately $30.00 to $35.00 per 100 test strips.

What to Watch Out For
Because the color change is so slight between a positive and negative result, good color vision is necessary.

What the Test Results Can Mean

A positive test, especially one confirmed by a positive urine **Nitrite** test, is sufficient to warrant medical consultation. If the positive tests are accompanied by any symptoms of a urinary tract infection, immediate medical attention should be sought. The test is also of value in following the course of treatment of a urinary tract infection.

NITRITE

Urine nitrite testing offers a reasonably accurate means of indicating the possibility of a urinary tract infection. It does not, however, ascertain the source or location of the infection; it could be in the kidneys, the ureters (the tiny tubes that carry urine from the kidneys to the bladder) or the bladder itself. At times the test can hint at an infection of the prostate or urethra (the tube that carries urine from the bladder to the outside). The test result depends on obtaining urine that has stayed in the bladder for several hours, allowing bacteria, if present, to act on dietary nitrates and change them to nitrites. Usually, the first morning specimen is best for testing. Because not all types of bacteria affect urine in the same way, the test is not an absolute one. When urinary tract infection is suspected, however, the test can help confirm the suspicions, and when used in conjunction with the urine **Leukocyte** test, the accuracy and significance of the test are increased.

The technique of collecting the urine is important; the clean-catch specimen (see the discussion of obtaining a clean-catch specimen in the urine testing introduction), with all its attendant cleansing, also helps ensure greater accuracy. The test is also employed to follow the success of treatment of urinary tract infections and to screen people, especially young children, who seem unusually susceptible to repeated infections.

What Is Usual

Normally urine is sterile; thus, the urine nitrite test result should be negative (show no evidence of nitrite that would be produced by urinary bacteria). If the total urine specimen is tested, as opposed to a clean-catch specimen, a slightly positive test may be obtained, due to the possibility of bacteria at the entrance to the urethra.

What You Need

A dipstick-type testing strip that includes the nitrite test; the N-Uristix is the least expensive, at approximately $14.00 for 100 test strips, and this strip also includes urine **Glucose** and **Protein** tests. The Multistix and the Chemstrip 8 include seven other tests and cost approximately $25.00 per 100 strips. The

Chemstrip 9 adds the **Leukocyte** test and costs a few pennies more per test.

A Microstix-Nitrite kit is also available; it includes three nitrite test dipsticks and three urine-collection cups and costs $3.55. The kit, which the manufacturer claims will detect 90 percent of all urinary infections, allows for three consecutive days of urine self-testing.

What to Watch Out For
The urine sample to be tested should have been in the bladder for at least four hours prior to testing.

• If you are taking large amounts of vitamin C and there is an excess of the vitamin in your urine (see Urine Tests, **Vitamin C** test), the test may show a false-negative result

• Urine that shows a very high result on the **Specific Gravity** test may also show a false-negative result when tested for nitrites

• If the urine specimen has been kept standing for more than 30 minutes before testing, a false-positive test may be observed.

What the Test Results Can Mean
A positive test usually indicates an infection somewhere in the urinary tract, but it is possible to have an infection and still show a negative test, depending on the causative bacteria. Your doctor can supply you with a special dipstick test called the Microstix-3, which requires a 24-hour incubation period; it can confirm your suspicions and also help identify the bacteria. Two consecutive positive nitrite tests, especially if confirmed by the urine **Leukocyte** test and the **Two/Three-Glass** test, warrant medical attention. A urinary tract infection can spread back up to the kidneys and become a very serious illness. When used to detect the possibility of a urinary tract infection in infants and children, a positive test and a medical consultation can help prevent complications in later life.

ODOR

While it is easy to imagine anyone's reluctance to test the aroma of urine, it should be kept in mind that long before the era of advanced medical technology, doctors not only routinely noted the scent of urine but tasted it as well as a means of diagnosis. And even today there are some doctors who request their patients to eat asparagus and make a note of the time it took before its characteristic odor appeared in the urine as a rough measure of kidney function. Many other foods and drugs affect the aromatic nature of urine but with insufficient consistency to indicate any diagnostic coincidence.

What Is Usual
Urine should have some odor, but it is usually not disagreeable; some people describe it as "spicy." If urine is left standing for a prolonged period of time, it usually acquires an ammonia–like odor.

What You Need
A clean, dry, container and normal smell function (see Brain and Nervous System Tests, **Smell Function** test).

What to Watch Out For
A container having any residual soap or detergent odors can disguise urine odors.

What the Test Results Can Mean
A sweet or fruity odor can mean:

- Diabetes (see Urine Tests, **Glucose** and **Ketones** tests); if you are on an Atkin's-type diet (eating few, or no, carbohydrates), the consequent production of acetone in urine can cause a similar odor
- A maple syrup odor, usually in infants, points to an inherited disorder actually called maple syrup disease.

A sour or otherwise unusual odor coming from an infant's urine can be an early warning signal of several other genetic metabolic disorders.

An ammonia-like or disagreeable odor in fresh urine hints at a urinary tract infection (see Urine Tests, **Nitrite** and **Leucocyte** tests).

Any persistent, unusual odor in urine warrants medical consultation.

pH

The pH of urine is an indication of its acidity or alkalinity; pH is usually measured by a number system, with 7 being neutral (that is, neither acid nor alkaline). Less than 7 is acid; greater than 7 is alkaline. Virtually every body activity—the quantity of fluids taken in, the metabolism of food, the amount of physical exertion and even one's emotional state—can alter the degree of acidity of urine.

The kinds of food one eats also influence urinary pH; large amounts of meat or fish in the diet, some fruits such as prunes and cranberries, or even a prolonged lack of food will usually cause an acid reaction. In contrast, eating most citrus fruits (which seem "acid"), along with most vegetables, will cause the urine to be alkaline. Dairy foods seem to prevent acidity in urine.

Some drugs can also alter urinary pH; vitamin C, ammonium chloride used as a diuretic and certain urinary antiseptics may make urine more acid, while antacids such as bicarbonates may make urine alkaline. There are certain drugs that need either an acid or an alkaline urine in order to work more efficiently. Urine pH can also help reflect whether many different body functions are normal. It is possible to help prevent and, in some instances, cure kidney stones by controlling the pH of the urine.

What Is Usual

Urine usually has a pH of about 6, or is slightly acid most of the time. It can normally range from 4.5 to 8, depending not only on diet but also on the time of day; it is usually more acid on awakening and more alkaline right after a meal. A good sign of normal kidney function is a pH that varies from 5 to 8 during a 24-hour period.

What You Need

The simplest and least expensive way to test urine pH is with litmus paper. While 100 separate acid and alkaline test strips cost about 80 cents, the result will only reveal acidity or alkalinity qualitatively; the strips do not indicate specific number values. The test can also be made with inexpensive chemicals such as those used to test swimming pool water, but these are usually difficult to work with and can be messy. The easiest way of obtaining number values for urine pH is through the multiple-dipstick test strips that also measure other urine values. The least expensive of these combine pH measurements along with glucose and protein testing. One is called Chemstrip 3; another is called Combistix. They cost from $12.00 to $15.00 for 100 test strips. Test strips that measure up to 10 different urine values, including pH, cost about $25.00 per 100.

What to Watch Out For
- Always keep in mind in performing this test the many different foods and drugs that can alter urine pH
- If you are taking drugs, ask your doctor or pharmacist about the possible effect they may have on urine pH
- Be sure the container used to collect the urine is clean and dry and has no soap or detergent residue that can affect pH
- Follow the test strip's directions carefully; some dipsticks require a specific waiting period before reading the test value
- Urine left standing for any length of time allows the growth of contaminating bacteria and may show a false-alkaline reaction; it may also give off an ammonia odor.

What the Test Results Can Mean

If you find you show an acid pH all the time, it could be from a metabolic condition such as diabetes, but it could also mean kidney trouble, heart or circulatory disease, a lung condition that interferes with proper transfer of oxygen from the lungs to the bloodstream or an infection somewhere in the body.

If you show an alkaline pH regularly, it could reflect stomach or intestinal difficulties, various hormone disorders, some nerve diseases and the possibility of anemia. Urinary tract infections may cause a persistent acid or alkaline urine, depending on the instigating bacteria.

Urine that is consistently either acid or alkaline warrants a medical consultation.

PHENYLKETONURIA SCREENING

Phenylketonuria (PKU) is an inherited metabolic disorder in which the body cannot properly metabolize the protein amino acid phenylalanine because of a genetic deficiency of an enzyme. The consequence of an excessive amount of phenylalanine in the body can be mental retardation. The disorder seems to occur once in every 10,000 births and is most common among people from northern Ireland and western Scotland; in the United States, approximately 300 infants are born each year with PKU. Throughout most of the United States, the blood or urine of newborn infants is required to be tested for phenylketonuria. But because of the increasing practice of home deliveries and mothers leaving the hospital a day or so after giving birth, the chance of missing the condition has increased. The test cannot be properly performed until sufficient milk protein has had the opportunity to be digested—a minimum of 24 hours (many experts say two weeks) after the infant has had its first formula-milk meal. Breast-fed infants must be tested again one month later.

The urine test for phenylpyruvic acid is only a screening test for PKU; it does not offer a definitive diagnosis. The test, however, can provide a valuable warning signal for pregnant women (large amounts of phenylalanine in a mother-to-be can damage the fetus), for relatives of patients with phenylketonuria and for infants who have unexplained convulsions or severe diaper rash, albeit they once tested negative for PKU. Many doctors recommend that every newborn be tested at home once a week until the infant is 6 weeks of age, in order to identify any infant in whom PKU might have been missed during hospital testing. The test is also performed to help parents evaluate the efficacy of dietary treatment for the disease.

Although this test is primarily intended for PKU screening, it has also been found to be of value in:

- Detecting abuse of certain tranquilizers (phenothiazine preparations such as Compazine, Phenergan, Sparine, Stelazine, Temeril, Thorazine and Vesprin)
- Detecting salicylate poisoning or abuse (aspirin is one form of salicylate).

What Is Usual
No trace of phenylpyruvic acid (the urine by-product of phenylalanine) should be detected in the urine or when the dipstick is pressed against a freshly wet diaper. A very small amount of phenylalanine seems necessary for normal growth, but children differ markedly as to how much they can eat, and properly metabolize, without showing symptoms of phenylketonuria.

What You Need
A dipstick-type test strip called Phenistix; they cost from $7.00 to $8.00 for a bottle of 50 strips.

What to Watch Out For
- Only freshly voided urine should be tested
- Do not test on disposable diapers; many have been manufactured with chemicals that can cause both false-positive and false-negative reactions
- If a greenish color appears, check the urine for bilirubin (see Urine Tests, **Bilirubin** test).

What the Test Results Can Mean
A positive test warrants immediate medical attention even though false-positive tests are frequent; blood phenylalanine measurements must be performed to confirm the diagnosis. The sooner a definitive diagnosis is made, the sooner dietary treatment can begin; early treatment can prevent mental retardation.

Negative tests should be repeated up to 6 weeks of age; a negative test in an infant with any suspicion of retardation, convulsions or eczema (severe rash) should not be considered definitive, and immediate medical attention is warranted.

Note: People who cannot metabolize phenylalanine should not use the artificial sugar substitute sweetener called aspartame (one brand name is NutraSweet; another is Equal).

Although the test can be performed on mothers-to-be who were once treated or are still being treated for phenylketonuria, it is necessary to have blood phenylalanine levels performed early in and throughout the pregnancy. A pregnant woman with elevated blood phenylalanine levels can not only harm her fetus by causing mental retardation; an excess of the amino acid can also cause congenital heart disease, and many other birth defects.

Drug Abuse

A positive test (color change) unrelated to phenylketonuria screening should make one think of an excessive use of certain tranquilizers, or aspirin and other salicylates. Children and the elderly, because of their metabolism, are much more susceptible to salicylate poisoning—especially if they have access to any of the hundreds of products containing aspirin, salicylates, salicylamide or salsalates. Some of the symptoms and signs of salicylate poisoning include: multiple black and blue bruises, confusion, disorientation, drowsiness, nausea and vomiting, ringing in the ears, difficulty in breathing, muscle twitchings, inappropriate sweating and flushed face, and a rapid heart rate and low blood pressure; at times such a person could be thought of as being drunk. Usually the Phenistix turns brownish-yellow with moderate salicylate poisoning and purple with a more severe overdose; any color change warrants medical attention.

PREGNANCY

Usually, once each month, halfway between menstrual periods, a fertile woman gives off an egg (ovum) from one of her ovaries. This is called ovulation time (see Miscellaneous Tests, **Body Temperature** test). The egg then starts its travels through the Fallopian tube to the uterus. If, during its passage, the egg meets sperm, it may become fertilized. If fertilized, it may then attach itself to the wall of the uterus through contact with specially formed cells that eventually become the placenta, and pregnancy occurs. Those cells, once implantation of the fertilized egg in the uterus takes place, start giving off a hormone called human chorionic gonadotropin (HCG). And it is the detection of this hormone in urine that is the basis for the pregnancy test. As pregnancy progresses, the amount of the hormone increases for the first two months; the usual home-type tests will not detect the hormone until at least a week after the missed menstrual period should have occurred, while certain intricate laboratory assays can pick up traces of the hormone within a week after conception (or even prior to when the menstrual period would have begun).

Pregnancy tests are performed not only to confirm an existing pregnancy but also are, or should be, performed before a woman of childbearing age has X-ray examinations or takes drugs—even some drugs that do not require a prescription. Only in this way can any adverse effects of radiation and medication on the fetus be avoided.

At least two dozen relatively rapid screening tests for pregnancy are available; most of these are sold to physicians for use in the office or to give to patients for use at home. Some slide-type tests can provide an answer within 90 seconds, but most tube-type tests take from one to two hours. Tube-type tests are usually more sensitive to smaller amounts of HCG. There are at least

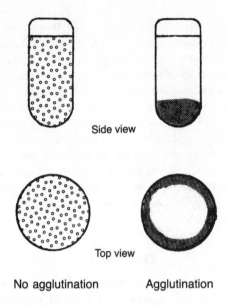

Side view

Top view

No agglutination   Agglutination

Figure 3. Drawing of agglutination, such as might be seen in certain urine pregnancy tests.

five different tests available without the need of a doctor's prescription. All the home tests are generally tube-type and contain HCG, usually attached to human or sheep red blood cells, and HCG antiserum from either humans, sheep or rabbits. The antiserum neutralizes most potentially interfering substances in the urine, and if a woman has been secreting her own HCG, she will also be manufacturing HCG antibodies. When HCG and HCG antibodies are present, they will combine with the blood cells and agglutinate or form a precipitation of granules at the bottom of a test tube. This is easily seen as a ring of particles settling as sediment. If no HCG is present, the blood cells remain in suspension, and no ring or clumping of particles is seen (Figure 3). Each home test comes with explicit, easy-to-follow directions. Always use the first morning urine specimen.

A great many drugs can cause a false-positive pregnancy test, and this must be kept in mind. A few examples include:

- Tranquilizers such as barbiturates, Compazine, Librium, Phenergan (also used as an antihistaminic or antiallergy medication), Stelazine, Thorazine and Valium
- Antibiotics such as penicillin, streptomycin, some sulfa preparations
- Pain relievers such as codeine, Darvon, Demerol, methadone and morphine

- Hormones such as cortisone preparations, estrogens, insulin, progesterone and thyroid
- Caffeine in excessive amounts.

A few of the special pregnancy tests supplied by doctors, however, will not show a false-positive reaction from drugs.

It is also possible to have a false-positive urine pregnancy test if your diet has included raw milk and after receiving certain vaccines for immunization; both can cause specific antibodies to form that react with the pregnancy test.

A urine specimen containing bacteria, blood or protein, or with a high specific gravity, may cause a false-positive test (see Urine Tests, **Nitrite**, **Blood**, **Protein** and **Specific Gravity** tests). A urine specimen with a very low specific gravity may not contain enough HCG to show up on the test.

What Is Usual
A positive test in the presence of pregnancy; a negative test where pregnancy does not exist. Some women in the menopause may show a false-positive test with certain types of pregnancy tests. Because so many drugs can cause a false-positive test, these must be taken into consideration before ascertaining that actual pregnancy exists. A negative test should be repeated one week later if there is any suspicion or fear of pregnancy.

What You Need
Home pregnancy test kits vary in price, claimed sensitivity, ease of use and time required. They include:

- *ACU-TEST*—takes one hour; manufacturer claims it can show a positive test, if pregnancy exists, nine days after last menstrual period was due; $10.00
- *ANSWER*—takes two hours; manufacturer claims it can show a positive test, if pregnancy exists, nine days after last menstrual period was due; $13.00
- *DAISY 2*—takes one hour; manufacturer claims it can show a positive test, if pregnancy exists, six days after last menstrual period was due; $15.00, but kit contains two tests
- *e.p.t.*—takes two hours; manufacturer claims it can show a positive test, if pregnancy exists, nine days after last menstrual period was due; $12.00 for one test kit, $18.00 for package of two test kits
- *PREDICTOR*—takes one hour; manufacturer claims it can show a positive test, if pregnancy exists, nine days after last menstrual period was due; $9.00.

Pregnancy tests supplied by doctors take from 90 seconds to two hours and are claimed to show a positive test, if pregnancy exists, just before or within a day or two after the last menstrual period was due. They cost the doctor from $1.00 to $2.00 per test.

You will also need a clean, dry container for the urine; any trace of soap, detergent or other contaminant can cause a false result. If possible, use a new, disposable plastic or wax cup.

What to Watch Out For
- Do not test urine that is more than one hour old; although many tests allow refrigeration of urine if there is to be a delay in testing, the older a urine specimen is, the less accurate the test
- Some of the tests require that the tube containing the urine and the chemical materials stay absolutely motionless during the test time; any bumping of the table or counter holding the tube or vibrations of the tube can cause a false result
- Do not place the tube in the sun or near any source of heat; it can cause a false result
- Do not attempt the test if the liquid in the tube is cloudy; the store will usually replace it without charge
- Be sure to follow the test's directions for interpreting the result; a positive result may look quite different with each different brand of test
- If you have any doubt about the color or condition of your urine before you start the test, perform urine **Blood**, **Nitrite**, **Protein** and **Specific Gravity** tests; pregnancy tests supplied by doctors usually overcome the effects of these interfering substances as well as most drugs; do not test yourself for pregnancy if your urine shows a positive test for blood, nitrite or protein; urine with a low specific gravity may not contain sufficient hormone and a false-negative test could result.

What the Test Results Can Mean
A negative pregnancy test, especially after a missed menstrual period, may have been performed too early to match the sensitivity of the test; repeat the test one week later. If still negative, in the face of a missed menstrual period, a medical consultation is warranted.

A positive pregnancy test most often means pregnancy; medical attention is warranted. It is never too early in pregnancy to start professional prenatal care. A positive test can, however, also come from many other conditions: Infections such as hepatitis have been known to cause positive results; various tumors of the ovary and uterus can cause a positive test; even menstrual irregularities may cause a positive test, albeit false. Thus, a positive pregnancy test warrants medical attention—if only to determine the cause if it is a false-positive result.

Note: Although home pregnancy tests can have a 98 percent accuracy rate, recent studies have shown that because of failure to follow test directions precisely, the accuracy rate is only about 75 percent.

PROTEIN

Urine testing is considered the best, easiest-to-perform home test for health evaluation, and the urine test for protein is probably the most valuable single urine examination. It is the best overall screening test for kidney disease and can also offer an early warning sign of heart and artery problems; liver, nerve and thyroid dysfunction; and even of hidden cancers and virus disease. As blood flows through the kidneys, a very tiny amount of protein is normally filtered out into the urine, but in such a minute quantity that it is usually not detectable through routine testing. Normal protein products in the blood consist primarily of albumins and globulins. Albumins help keep a proper chemical-to-plasma balance in the blood; they also attach themselves to hormones, enzymes, vitamins and drugs and carry them throughout the body to provide nutrition for cells and assist in their metabolic functions. Globulins help transport immune substances throughout the body to fight off infections and other diseases.

The use of many different drugs, certain foods (such as an excessive intake of protein), irritants like mustard, exposure to chemical poisons, strenuous physical exercise, being chilled, and even extreme anxiety or discomfort can cause a temporary positive protein test reaction, and all these nondisease factors must be taken into account when testing urine for protein.

What Is Usual
Although some doctors dismiss an occasional trace of detectable protein in the urine, the general consensus is that unless there is a good explanation for its being there (exercise, cold, use of certain antibiotics or some sleeping medicines, etc.), there should never be any measurable protein in the urine. And if protein should be detected, it should only be observed temporarily; it should not persist. There is a condition known as orthostatic albuminuria, in which a few people show protein in the urine whenever they are standing for a period of time—such as when playing golf—but the protein should be completely absent when the urine is tested after the individual has been lying down for a few hours. For home testing, however, it is best to consider urine as being totally protein-free.

What You Need
The easiest way to test for urine protein is with a dipstick-type plastic strip. Strips for protein testing only are available as Albustix, for about $9.00 per hundred test strips. The Combistix GP, which also include glucose testing

along with protein, sell for about the same price. Most multiple-test dipsticks include protein as one component and cost about $25.00 per hundred strips.

There are other ways to test for urine protein:

- One is to place the urine in a heatproof test tube and warm the upper portion of the urine in the tube over a flame for a few seconds. If protein is present, the upper portion of the urine sample will congeal or cloud up, much like the cooked white of an egg, while the lower portion of the sample will remain clear (Figure 4).
- Another way is to add about one teaspoon of white vinegar slowly down the side of the tube (or glass) into the urine and look for clouding.
- The Bumintest tablets (a form of sulfosalicylic acid) offers a very accurate test as well as a check on dipstick results; they cost $50.00 for 100 tablets. Usually, four tablets are dissolved in one ounce of water and each ounce of solution will perform 45 to 50 tests.

What to Watch Out For
A false-positive test can come from:

- Residual cleaning substances in the container
- Any contamination of the urine specimen (menstruation, vaginal discharge, a prostate infection, sexual activity)
- An alkaline urine (see Urine Tests, **pH** test)
- Recent X-rays over the abdomen
- The use of certain drugs
- The test strip being old or having been exposed to air, light or heat for a period of time.

Be sure to observe the strict time limitations stipulated in the test's directions, and only read the color changes if you have normal color vision.

What the Test Results Can Mean
Proteinuria, as protein in the urine is called, can come from:

- Kidney disease and urinary tract conditions such as bladder infection
- Sexually transmitted diseases
- High blood pressure, not necessarily due to kidney involvement
- Other forms of heart and artery disease
- Diabetes and certain other hormone imbalances
- Infections—no matter where they are in the body
- Several different forms of cancer
- Some very rare conditions such as lupus erythematosus or amyloidosis.

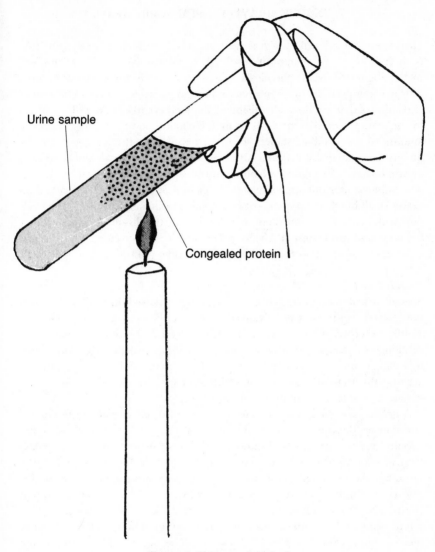

Urine sample

Congealed protein

Figure 4. Urine protein test.

Thus, the finding of protein in the urine on more than one occasion, especially when there seems to be no known or obvious nondisease cause, warrants medical consultation, even if only to rule out a defective test strip. Because persistent proteinuria may be an early warning sign of kidney or heart disease, such a test finding justifies the ruling out of any potential disease process as soon as possible.

SPECIFIC GRAVITY (and Mosenthal Test)

Measurement of the specific gravity of urine is a reflection of its density; that is, an indication of the amount of solid material dissolved in the urine specimen being tested. Many chemicals such as sodium chloride grains (salt), urea nitrogen compounds, sugar molecules, protein particles, calcium, phosphates and sulfates that are normally dissolved in blood are filtered out of the blood by the kidneys and become virtually invisible matter in urine. The greater the amount of dissolved substances in the urine solution, the higher its specific gravity. In a normal individual eating and drinking a typical American diet, approximately 450 gallons of blood flow through the kidneys every 24 hours. The kidneys filter out approximately 45 gallons of plasma each day and then reabsorb all but 1 to 1:5 quarts of fluid, which ultimately end up in the bladder. With urination, a portion of urine containing the dissolved material leaves the body and can be tested. Urine specific gravity measurements are but one of several indications as to the ability of the kidneys to function properly.

What Is Usual
Specific gravity is reported as a numerical figure based on the fact that distilled water, containing no dissolved solids, would show a relative value of 1.000; therefore, the more solid matter dissolved in solution, the higher the resulting number. Single urine specific gravity values usually range from 1.010 to 1.025, assuming a typical diet, typical fluid intake and moderate physical activity; throughout a 24-hour day, different measurements should show a variation of at least 0.010 in two or more samples.

A normal specific gravity measurement can also reflect many different circumstances: the time of day (after a night's sleep, without food or fluids, the specific gravity is greater and shows a higher reading than after routine daytime activities and diet); the quantity and quality of foods and fluids (the more liquids consumed, the more dilute the urine and the lower the specific gravity reading); excessive physical activity (when body water is lost through perspiration, there is less of it to pass through the kidneys, resulting in a less-dilute urine and a higher specific gravity reading). Thus, a single measurement ranging from 1.005 to 1.035 could still be normal, depending on the circumstances.

What You Need
The most common test apparatus to determine urine specific gravity is a hydrometer (frequently called a urinometer when sold primarily for urinalysis). It is a small, weighted glass float with a numerical scale that indicates how deep the float sinks into the liquid being tested. The scale usually reads from 1.000 to 1.060; the greater the amount of dissolved material, the less the float sinks and the higher the specific gravity reading (Figure 5). A hydrometer

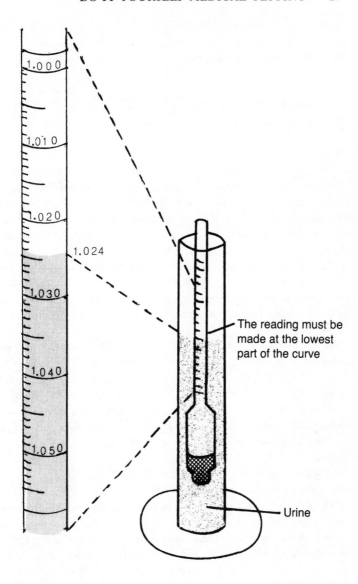

Figure 5. Urine specific gravity test, as measured by a urinometer (hydrometer).

(urinometer) ranges in cost from $3.00 to $5.00, depending on its size, and usually comes with a tall glass tube in which to place the hydrometer; the smaller size is quite adequate for urine testing. For repeated measurements this is the least expensive equipment.

The newest and simplest technique for testing urine specific gravity utilizes a thin strip of chemically treated paper that is dipped into a urine sample; the color change is compared with a chart to give specific gravity values. The plastic dip-and-test strips (N-Multistix-SG) for specific gravity are part of comprehensive dipsticks that also include eight other urine tests on the same strip; they cost from $27.00 to $30.00 for a package of 100 strips, or about 27 to 30 cents a test.

What to Watch Out For

Although routine testing of urine for specific gravity has no adverse effects, measurements that involve evaluating the concentration and dilution of urine following excessive intake and then deprivation of fluids should not be undertaken if there is the slightest suspicion of kidney disease, except under a doctor's supervision. At such times it could be dangerous to deprive the kidneys of fluid.

As a general check on the accuracy of urine specific gravity measurements, a high specific gravity is usually found in urine with a deep amber or orange color; in contrast, the lower the specific gravity, the lighter yellow and clearer the urine color. An inconsistency between specific gravity and color can point to disease.

When using a hydrometer it is important to have sufficient urine in the glass testing cylinder to ensure that the hydrometer floats freely and that it does not touch the sides of the tube. The hydrometer must be kept scrupulously clean. The reading should come from the lowest part of the level of the curve formed by the top of the liquid against the scale. Urinary hydrometers must be checked for accuracy regularly (by placing the hydrometer in distilled water, where it should read 1.000), as they frequently become erroneous.

If a urine specimen also contains abnormal amounts of sugar, protein or other chemicals, the specific gravity readings will be abnormally high, and the effect of such substances must be taken into account to obtain a correct reading. If you do know the amount of glucose or protein in the urine to be tested, (see Urine Tests, **Glucose** and **Protein** tests) a general rule of thumb is to subtract 0.003 from the observed reading for every one gram of glucose or protein per 100 ml of urine (3.5 ounces). If a patient has been taking diuretic drugs, the specific gravity reading will be low as a result of the excessive amount of fluid the drugs prevent the kidneys from reabsorbing.

What the Test Results Can Mean

When urine specific gravity shows a value of from 1.015 to 1.030 in the first specimen voided that day, and assuming no food or drink intake for the previous eight hours, it is usually a reasonable indication that the kidneys are capable of concentrating urine normally. Additionally evidence of normal kidney function would be a specific gravity measurement of from 1.007 to

1.020 in the evening, especially after normal food and drink intake during the day, showing the kidneys' ability to dilute the urine when appropriate. An occasional deviation from what would be expected is not necessarily an abnormal result, especially when hydration, physical activity and diet are taken into account. It is the repeated observation of unexpected, abnormal values that points to a kidney malfunction or some hormone imbalance.

As an example of how the specific gravity test can hint at hormone activity (as long as all other kidney function tests are normal), when an individual is subjected to unusual stress—especially of an emotional nature—or pressure, the specific gravity may read as high as 1.040. Anxiety-producing situations can cause an antidiuretic hormone (ADH) known as vasopressin to be manufactured in greater-than-normal amounts. This hormone slows down urine excretion from the kidneys, and the fluid that does filter through becomes very concentrated. Some doctors use this test as a means of evaluating a patient's response to provocation (also see Miscellaneous tests, Vitamin C Body Level).

Another antidiuretic hormone appraisal includes the repeated observation of urine with a high specific gravity accompanied by an unexplained bad temper, confusion, and sometimes convulsions and coma. This can, at times, come from the "syndrome of inappropriate antidiuretic hormone secretion" (SIADH), and while it may be brought on as a consequence of cancer, severe infections and many other diseases, it can also occur as a side effect of many medicines, especially diuretic drugs. The discovery of this syndrome can be a warning signal to search for some undetected disorder.

Diseases of the parathyroid gland that prevent the kidneys from excreting normal amounts of calcium in the urine can result in extremely low urine specific gravity measurements; taking too much vitamin D can also cause similar test results. And when amounts of urine voided reach from 10 to 20 quarts a day, along with specific gravity measurements of 1.007 or less, it is a fairly reliable indication of diabetes insipidus, a rare disease in which the pituitary gland fails to manufacture sufficient vasopressin—the antidiuretic hormone. While the condition can be inherited, it can also occur after a head injury or subsequent to severe generalized infections.

If abnormal specific gravity measurements persist or do not correspond with usual patterns of eating, drinking and other physical activity, the test could be an early warning sign of some impending disease process. A particularly ominous observation is specific gravity measurements that stay close to the same number value at all times. Repeated abnormal specific gravity measurements are sufficient reason to seek medical attention.

The Mosenthal Test
The specific gravity test's principal purpose is to assist, along with several other related tests, in the evaluation of kidney function and to aid in locating that part of the kidney that might be malfunctioning. One way of doing this

is to assess the kidneys' ability to concentrate the urine under controlled conditions—sometimes called the Mosenthal test, which is performed as follows:

Drink no liquids (usual solid foods are permitted) for 24 hours prior to testing. Then, on awakening in the morning, test the urine for specific gravity. Return to bed and stay as relaxed as possible for another hour and then test a second urine specimen for specific gravity. Following the second test, get up and be active for one more hour (eat or drink nothing during the test), and test a third urine specimen for specific gravity. At least one of the three urine samples tested should show a specific gravity of 1.025 or higher as an indication that the kidneys can concentrate urine when liquids are withheld. If all three samples show a specific gravity of less than 1.020, medical consultation is warranted for more specific kidney evaluation. Again, this test should not be performed when there is the slightest suspicion of kidney disease except under a doctor's observation.

TURBIDITY

The turbidity of urine is a reflection of its cloudiness. Cloudy urine most often comes from an excess of certain minerals, particularly phosphates, but many other substances can contribute to turbidity: pus, blood, bacteria, parasites, proteins and even fats can, at times, be found in urine.

What Is Usual
Urine should be clear, especially immediately after urination. If a urine sample is left standing for a prolonged period of time, it may appear cloudy but not be unusual.

What You Need
A clear glass container.

What to Watch Out For
Do not use a container that might have any residue of soap or detergent. If you are a woman with a vaginal discharge, it could make clear urine appear turbid. A man's urine may appear cloudy after sexual activity.

What the Test Results Can Mean
Continuous cloudy urine could be an early warning signal of kidney stones and deserves medical consultation. It could also indicate a urinary tract infection, and if the urine **Nitrite** and **Leukocyte** tests are also positive, medical attention is indicated. Some rare causes of turbidity include diabetes, filariasis (a parasitic invasion of the body), a lymph system problem, a sexually transmitted disease or a tumor somewhere within the body.

TWO/THREE-GLASS

When, while urinating, the urine is voided into separate containers, the very first portion of urine (about a teaspoon) that is voided into the first glass carries with it any substances that lay within the urethra—that portion of the urinary system that starts at the bladder and ends at the point where the urine leaves the body. It can contain material from an infectious process in the urethra (see Urine Tests, **Nitrite** test) such as gonorrhea or chlamydia, as well as white blood cells (see Urine Tests, **Leukocyte** test) that usually respond to an infectious process. The major portion of urine is then voided into a second glass and consists of what has been stored in the bladder. Just prior to the termination of urination, the last remaining bit of urine may be voided into a third glass in order to help confirm, or reveal, a beginning bladder infection or, in men, a prostate problem. An optional refinement of the three-glass test, in men, is to stop urination just prior to emptying the bladder completely and have the prostate examined; the third glass can then better reflect prostatic involvement. Thus, by observing the turbidity (cloudiness) and color (see Urine Tests, **Turbidity** and **Color** tests) in the two or three containers, it is sometimes possible to locate the specific area of a urinary tract problem.

What Is Usual
The urine in the two or three containers should be clear and even sparkling. The color should be light yellow (straw-colored), and there should be no turbidity (Figure 6).

What You Need
Two or three clear glass containers, one capable of holding at least one pint. Although this test can be performed at any time of the day, the first morning specimen is best. Void a small quantity of urine into the first container and, if the two-glass test is being performed, all the rest into the large container. If the three-glass test is to be conducted, the last teaspoon should be voided into the third container. In men urination may be stopped just before the bladder feels empty and then, after a brief prostate examination, concluded (see Genitourinary System Tests, **Prostate Observations**).

What to Watch Out For
Any contamination in the glass containers that might cause cloudiness in the urine. Do not massage or apply pressure to the penis during this test.

What the Test Results Can Mean
If the small amount of urine collected in the first container is cloudy and the second portion less cloudy, it usually signifies a urethral infection, possibly a sexually transmitted disease; it warrants medical attention. Should the first

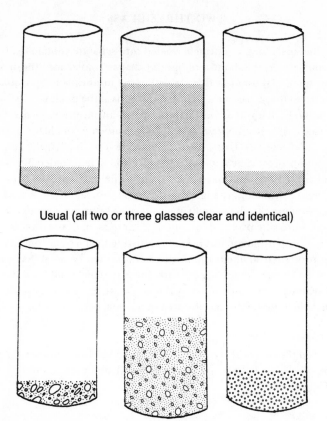

Usual (all two or three glasses clear and identical)

Abnormal (first container most cloudy, decreasing in next one or two; usually from a urethral infection)

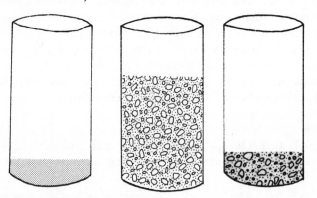

Abnormal (cloudiness increases in second or third container; usually from kidney, bladder or prostate infection)

Figure 6. Two (or three) glass urine test.

container show clear urine and the second show cloudy urine, there is the possibility of a bladder or kidney infection; it warrants medical consultation. The possibility of a urinary tract infection can also be confirmed by other urine tests (**Leukocyte, Nitrite, Protein**). Should both containers appear equally cloudy, and should the other urine tests indicate a possible infection, medical attention should be sought. When the third glass is tested, it should always be clear (or clearer than the other two); otherwise medical consultation is indicated.

Each of the two or three containers can also be tested for blood (see Urine Tests, **Blood** test); a positive result in one of the glasses warrants medical attention and may indicate the area of the genito-urinary system involved (Figure 7).

URINE FLOW RATE (Uroflowmetry)

The peak urinary flow rate is really a measure of the greatest force of the urinary stream achieved during urination and, by reflecting the pressure behind the urinary flow, it can sometimes indicate an obstruction in or narrowing of the urethra the duct that carries urine from the bladder to the outside (Figure 7). The test can also provide an early warning sign of problems that can affect the spinal cord and nerves to and from the bladder. Urine flow rate measurements are usually performed after symptoms attributable to the urinary tract are noticed: increased frequency of urination; the urge to void more than five times during the day with usual fluid intake; sudden, abrupt stopping of the urine flow for a moment or two during urination; a noticeable loss of force while urinating; a noticeable thinning of the urinary stream, pain while urinating. The test can also be performed on individuals without any relevant complaints. It is particularly valuable in following the response to treatment used to relieve any obstruction of urinary flow.

What Is Usual
The urinary flow rate is measured in milliliters per second (ml/sec); it takes 28 ml to make an ounce. The rate also depends on the volume, or how much urine is passed at one time; the greater the amount, the higher the flow rate. Women average from 8 to 32 ml/sec. With men, the age must be taken into account; older men usually have a lesser flow rate, but in general it averages from 10 to 36 ml/sec. The most important observation is to have no great or unexpected change over a period of time—say, every six months.

What You Need
A Peakometer (Figure 8), the brand name for a disposable urine flow meter made by the Kendall Company. It costs approximately $5.00 to $6.00, and though it is a disposable unit, it can be reused as a collection device for other

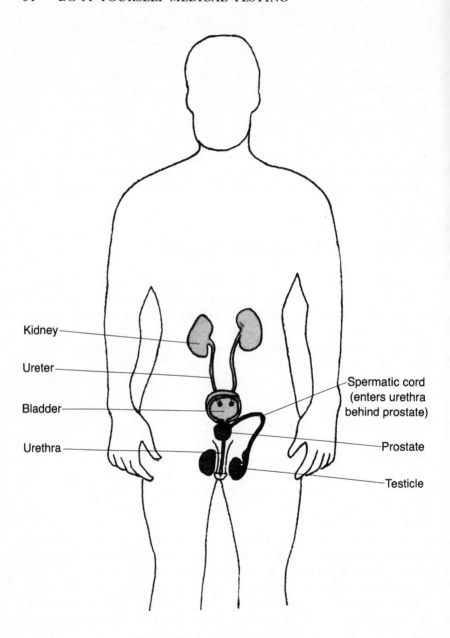

Figure 7. Male genitourinary system.

(The female urinary system is similar; the urethra is shorter and, obviously, there is no prostate, spermatic cord or testicle.)

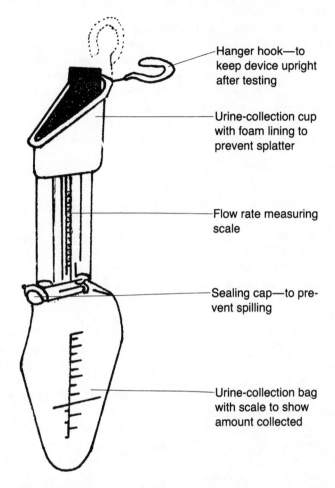

Hanger hook—to keep device upright after testing

Urine-collection cup with foam lining to prevent splatter

Flow rate measuring scale

Sealing cap—to prevent spilling

Urine-collection bag with scale to show amount collected

Figure 8. Urine flow rate, as measured by a peakometer, a urine flow rate measuring device.

urine tests. Simple instructions and record forms that take into account sex, age and the amount of urine produced accompany the meter.

What to Watch Out For
Strict adherence to the instructions—especially the warning not to shake, tilt or lay the device down, but to hang it on its accompanying hook immediately after use. Failure to drink enough fluids to allow proper measurements; it is best to drink four glasses of water about four hours before performing the test. Unless you urinate at least five ounces, the test will be invalid. Do not strain or force the urine flow.

What the Test Results Can Mean
Any reduced peak urinary flow rate, when charted on the accompanying patient record form, could come from an old urethral infection (sexually transmitted disease), prostate infection or enlargement, kidney stones, tumors (most likely in the bladder) and any of a number of nerve conditions such as multiple sclerosis or the consequences of nerve injuries. Although results from only one test should not be considered definitive, repeated below-normal peak urinary flow rates warrant medical attention. As with most diseases, the sooner treatment of a urinary tract obstruction is begun, the easier and more effective it is.

UROBILINOGEN

Urobilinogen is formed in the intestine from bilirubin, a yellow pigment that is part of the liver's bile (see Urine Tests, **Bilirubin** test). Very minute amounts are filtered from blood by the kidneys and can be detected in urine. For some unknown reason, afternoon urine—collected between 1:00 and 3:00 p.m.— contains the greatest concentration of urobilinogen, and when looking for this specific substance, midafternoon is the best time for testing. As with so many other urine tests, the taking of certain drugs, such as those used to treat gout and especially antibiotics, can cause false-negative values. At times the use of aspirin products can cause a false-positive result. Unlike many other urine tests, the absence of any urobilinogen in the urine can be as important as an excess. Because urobilinogen is one of the many end products of the breakdown of red blood cells, its presence can reflect certain anemias, especially those that come from red cell destruction. Its presence in more than trace amounts can also signal liver disease. Although the test can be performed by itself, it is more accurate when accompanied by the urine **Bilirubin** test as a substantiating check.

What Is Usual
It is considered normal to show no more than a trace of urobilinogen in urine, especially when the test is performed in the afternoon or on a sample collected over a 24-hour period.

What You Need
Although there are many chemical tests for urobilinogen, the easiest is one of the dipstick methods. A single-test strip for urobilinogen called the Urobilistix is available at $9.00 for 50 strips, but it is better to use one of the dipsticks that also incorporate bilirubin—usually along with several other tests— such as Multistix or Chemstrip 7, which cost approximately $22.00 for 100 test strips.

What to Watch Out For
- The urine to be tested must be freshly voided
- It must not be too acid, or a false-negative result can occur; if the urine is too alkaline, a false-positive result can occur. This is another reason why a multiple-test strip incorporating pH testing is more accurate (see urine **pH** test)
- The test strips must be fresh and not have been subjected to heat or moisture
- Any drug use that could interfere with the test must be noted (check with your doctor or pharmacist)
- Although a very low urobilinogen level may be detected, a negative test is not sensitive enough to indicate an absolute absence of urobilinogen
- You must have normal color vision.

What the Test Results Can Mean
Increased levels of urobilinogen usually mean liver or bile duct disease (any condition that prevents urobilinogen from being reabsorbed into the liver). Some other generalized infections such as mononucleosis (see Blood Tests, **Mononucleosis** test) can cause an elevated urine urobilinogen level. Prolonged constipation and some forms of heart disease that slow the circulation may also cause a positive test. While a few forms of anemia can also raise urobilinogen in the urine, the test is not specific enough to warrant anything but a medical consultation if any increase is noted; when performed with a urine **Bilirubin** test, it can help to distinguish liver disease from a blood problem.

VITAMIN C

Because of an ancient, genetically transmitted defect, the human is one of very few mammals that cannot manufacture its own vitamin C (ascorbic acid). And although this vitamin is not stored in large amounts in the body, it is still essential to the body's defense mechanisms (resistance to all forms of disease) and to the formation of bones and teeth. With a fairly normal diet, an individual usually ingests sufficient amounts of vitamin C to take care of the body's needs on a day-to-day basis; the addition of supplementary vitamins (commonly in pill form) more than makes up for any daily deficiency—unless, of course, you are a follower of the theory that humans need far greater amounts of ascorbic acid than is presently recommended by most nutritionists. People who do take massive or megadoses of vitamin C inevitably spill any excess not utilized by the body into their urine, and large amounts of vitamin C in the urine can cause:

- A false-positive urine **Glucose** test
- A false-positive urine **Blood** test
- A false-negative urine **Nitrite** test
- An abnormally high acidity result on the urine **pH** test.

Thus, this test is primarily of value when utilized to ascertain the accuracy of other urine tests; it can, of course, also indicate an absence of vitamin C in urine, but this test alone does not necessarily mean the individual has a definite vitamin C deficiency (scurvy). See Miscellaneous Tests, **Vitamin C Body Level.**

What Is Usual
Most healthy people on a balanced diet will excrete about 20 mg of ascorbic acid when measured in all urine passed over a 24-hour period. The amount may vary from a trace to 10 mg per 100 ml in a single urine specimen; and on occasion, depending on diet, a urine sample may show 40 mg per 100 ml or more at one time. When large amounts of vitamin C are taken, the test may show proportionately large amounts in the urine.

What You Need
A dipstick called C-STIX, which costs from $8.00 to $10.00 for a bottle of 50 sticks.

What to Watch Out For
- The test must be performed on freshly voided urine; urine that has been left standing for more than 15 minutes may give false-negative values
- The timing of the test is important; follow the test directions explicitly
- If the original color on the dipstick does not match the "O" on the accompanying color chart before use, or does not match the "O" when dipped in distilled water, do not use that bottle of dipsticks
- Certain drugs can cause false-positive reactions; check with your doctor or pharmacist if you are using any medicine.

What the Test Results Can Mean
Large amounts of vitamin C in the urine usually interfere with other urine tests and make urine test results for blood, glucose, nitrite and pH inaccurate; medical consultation is warranted if, after going without vitamin C for three days.

Very low, or no, vitamin C in the urine can mean an anemia, especially in an infant who is fed nothing but milk, and can also accompany infection, alcoholism and hiatal hernia (in which a portion of the stomach extends back up through the diaphragm and can cause an indigestion type of heartburn; see Gastrointestinal System Tests, **String** test). Some people with cancer show a very low level of vitamin C, even with a normal diet and vitamin C supplements. Repeated results showing no, or very little, vitamin C warrant medical consultation.

VOLUME

How much urine an individual passes in a 24-hour period can be as important an observation as any chemical reaction. Many diseases can first manifest their presence by either increasing or decreasing the amount of urine; alterations in one's nutritional state can also affect urine volume. And nocturia, or the need to urinate frequently during the night, can be an early-warning sign of several disorders.

What Is Usual
The average person, on a fairly typical diet of food and drink, usually passes from one to two quarts of urine in a 24-hour period. It is common to void from 6 to 8 ounces of urine at a time, with the exception being the first morning specimen on awakening, which averages 10 to 12 ounces. It is not unusual for a woman to have a decreased amount of urine for several days prior to menstruation and to have an increased volume for a few days after menstruation begins.

What You Need
A wide–mouthed container with ounce markings on the side. (An easy-to-use, inexpensive urine-collection measuring device is described in the **Urine Flow Rate** test.)

What to Watch Out For
- Be sure to take into account the amount and kinds of fluid you drink prior to, and during, the time you measure your urine volume; a large quantity of liquid taken in can cause a compensatory increase in urine output, and even small amounts of alcoholic beverages can disproportionately increase urine volume
- Cold weather can cause an increase in urine amounts (the kidneys handle the body fluid that is usually lost through perspiration), while warm weather or prolonged physical activity can reduce urine output
- Do not attempt to measure urine volume if you are taking any form of diuretic drug, are using salt substitutes or are under a doctor's care until you have discussed the test with your doctor.

What the Test Results Can Mean
If, after all the things that can cause increased or decreased urination have been taken into account, the 24-hour urine volume is repeatedly greater than two quarts a day, it could mean:

* Diabetes mellitus—the kind of diabetes that comes from the inability to metabolize carbohydrates; sometimes called sugar diabetes
* Diabetes insipidus—the kind of diabetes that comes from an inadequately produced brain hormone; sometimes called water diabetes
* Kidney disease
* A reflection of several different hormone imbalances
* Some form of metabolic disorder or deliberate starvation
* An indirect consequence of a psychological problem, usually accompanied by an increased fluid intake.

If the 24-hour urine volume is less than 16 ounces (one pint), it could mean:

* Kidney disease
* Heart disease
* An intestinal obstruction
* A reflection of a hormone imbalance.

Repeated urine volume increases or the increased need to urinate often (especially during the night), warrant medical consultation. An unexplainable decrease in urine volume requires immediate medical attention.

BLOOD TESTS

The analysis of the chemicals and other constituents of blood has long been the key to helping diagnose illness and searching for early warning signs of impending disease. The College of American Pathologists, whose members make up the majority of laboratory directors, claim there are now more than 850 different analytical procedures that can be performed on a blood sample.

Blood carries oxygen, enzymes, hormones and essential nutrients to all parts of the body; it also carries away carbon dioxide and other waste products of metabolism to the lungs, kidneys and skin. Thus, when something goes wrong anywhere in the body, cellular and/or chemical changes can occur in the blood, reflecting a disease or disorder. When tests are performed to study the red and white blood cells or platelets, such testing is usually referred to as *hematology*; when testing is limited to electrolytes, enzymes, fats, gases, hormones, minerals, proteins and protein products, sugars or organ products such as from the liver, it is usually referred to as *blood chemistry studies*.

Although blood is composed of a great many substances, for testing purposes it is separated into four categories:

- Whole blood—this includes all the cellular material, red and white blood cells, along with platelets (thrombocytes) and fibrinogen (for clotting), and the serum or liquid portion as well. (Fingertip blood is an example of whole blood)
- Cellular material alone
- Serum—the clear liquid portion of the blood after it has clotted and the clot (consisting of all cellular material) has been removed
- Plasma—the pale yellow liquid that remains after blood is collected in a container containing an anticoagulant (heparin or special chemical compound to prevent clotting); the cellular material, less the fibrinogen, is removed through centrifugation or by allowing the blood to stand while the solid elements settle to the bottom.

Most clinical laboratories test either serum or plasma because the chemical composition of blood cells tends to be more inconsistent; and for certain tests only serum can be used. In performing home blood testing, however, only whole blood is used; it is sufficiently stable and accurate for this purpose.

OBTAINING A BLOOD SAMPLE

What You Need

- A sterile needle or lancet; those who prefer a needle commonly use a 25-gauge, one-inch-long hypodermic or syringe-style needle; it is best to use individually wrapped, presterilized, disposable needles, which cost from 5 to 8 cents each
- Most people prefer disposable lancets that let you control the depth of penetration; one commercial brand is called Monolets, which cost about 5 cents each; these lancets can also be used with automatic (push-button) pricking devices such as the Autolet, which costs approximately $25.00; or the Autoclix, which costs approximately $20.00; or the Penlet, which looks like a small ball-point pen and costs approximately $10.00; such devices really do help eliminate much of the anxiety and discomfort of trying to stick oneself
- Gauze pads or cotton plus rubbing alcohol, or readily available, individually wrapped, alcohol-soaked "swabs," "prep-pads" or Zephirin towelettes, which cost $2.00 per 100.

Where to Stick

There are four areas where a drop of blood is easily obtained. They include:

- The fingertip—the most common site (either the index, middle or ring finger); if you make the puncture just slightly to the side of the center of the tip, it is reportedly less painful; (some people find that pressing the thumbnail hard against the fingertip to be punctured also lessens the discomfort)
- The soft portion of the earlobe—said to be the least painful area of all. If the earlobe is used, it is usually possible to collect additional drops of blood for additional or repeat tests from the one puncture site without the need for resticking by simply flicking the earlobe with the fingertip
- The back of the heel—supposedly the easiest site to obtain a drop of blood from young children
- Alongside the tip of the big toe—also used mostly with children.

What to Do

- Wash the area well with soap and water, then dry
- Rub the selected site with an alcohol-soaked gauze pad or "swab" and let the alcohol evaporate before making the puncture

- Make a small puncture hole with the needle or lancet
- Wipe away the first drop of blood that appears with a piece of sterile gauze or cotton
- Use the next full drop of blood for the test
- After the blood sample has been obtained, hold a piece of sterile gauze or cotton to the puncture site for a few minutes until the bleeding stops.

What to Watch Out For
- Do not puncture an area that is swollen or seems infected
- Be sure the puncture site is warm; warm it by applying warm cloths or soaking in warm water just before washing
- Be careful not to squeeze or milk puncture area to try to force bleeding; this can dilute the blood sample with fluids from adjacent tissues and cause a false test result
- Never use a needle that has been used by someone else or even one that has been sterilized by boiling; there is always the risk of transmitting hepatitis this way
- Avoid puncturing the same area repeatedly
- Never use any material if there is the slightest doubt about its sterility
- If testing someone else's blood, do not touch the blood sample; it could carry an infection
- Some blood tests require precision measurements; do not attempt such tests if you cannot be exacting in your technique.

Most people find that when a blood sample is to be obtained for the first time, it is best to perform the task in front of a doctor; this not only lends reassurance to the technique but assures a properly obtained blood sample.

Reporting Blood Test Results
Depending upon the type of test, blood values may be expressed in many different ways. Most chemical determinations are reported in milligrams per 100 milliliters (deciliters) or mg per 100 ml. This is an arbitrary measurement, indicating how much of a chemical would be found if 100 ml (3.5 ounces) of blood were evaluated; obviously only a minute amount of blood is examined, and so the 100 ml was chosen for standardization. Blood glucose and hemoglobin results are reported this way, although it is not unusual to report only the milligram amount as a solitary numerical figure (e.g., a blood sugar level of 110 mg per 100 ml would be reported simply as 110). Clotting time is reported in seconds of time, and many other tests to determine merely if a substance is present or not—such as for sickle-cell hemoglobin—are reported as positive, if present, and negative, if undetectable.

BLEEDING AND CLOTTING TIME

Although they are two essentially different tests, bleeding time and clotting time are usually tested together as a crude measure of how quickly bleeding will be stopped by normal body responses—a process called hemostasis. More specifically, bleeding time reflects the condition of the blood vessels—particularly the smallest ones called capillaries—by measuring how well they constrict and close off following an injury. Bleeding time also indicates how well the blood's platelets (tiny cells that clump together to plug the broken capillary) are performing. Clotting time, on the other hand, is a generalized indication of the performance of all the other body chemicals that contribute to clotting: antihemophilic substances, enzymes, minerals (calcium), proteins (prothrombin, the specific clotting factor disabled when anticoagulant drugs are prescribed).

The two tests offer screening information to help detect bleeding tendencies, whether inherited or resulting from anemia, lead poisoning, liver disease, cancer or radiation exposure; the use of drugs such as adrenalin, aspirin, some antibiotics, oral contraceptives, coumarin products (warfarin), phenylbutazone (for arthritis), cortisone preparations; or dietary deficiencies of calcium and vitamin K. The tests are especially valuable prior to medical or dental surgery and before prescribing certain drugs for a prolonged period of time.

Another test that can suggest a bleeding tendency but does not require sticking the finger to obtain blood is the **Capillary Fragility** test (see Heart and Circulation Tests); it primarily measures the strength of the capillary walls and whether or not sufficient platelets are present.

What Is Usual
If you stick your fingertip with a lancet or needle and, with clean blotting paper or gauze, gently remove the drops of blood as they appear, the bleeding should stop after ½ minute and before 3 minutes; this is a measure of bleeding time. If, on the other hand, you put that drop of blood on a clean glass slide or dish and touch it with a pin every 30 seconds, you should see evidence of a clot (a thin, sticky thread stuck to the pin) sometime between 6 and 16 minutes. A thin glass capillary tube may also be used; when you touch an open end of such a tube to a drop of blood, the blood automatically rises up into the tube by capillary action. Then, simply break a segment of the capillary tube periodically, starting at one end until you see evidence of a clot (a thin thread of blood remaining between the two pieces of broken glass) sometime between 6 and 16 minutes; this is the clotting time.

What You Need
One or more drops of blood (see Blood Tests, **Obtaining a Blood Sample**); some blotting paper (see Blood Tests, **Hemoglobin** test) or gauze pads; a few

plain microhematocrit capillary tubes, which cost from $1.50 to $2.00 for 100; and a watch or clock.

What to Watch Out For
Be sure the needle or lancet is sterile and that the blotting paper or gauze is clean or sterile. Keep in mind that any medicine you are taking can alter the test results; check with your doctor or pharmacist to see if your drugs can interfere with the test (even a few aspirin a day can double your bleeding time).

What the Test Results Can Mean
A prolonged bleeding and/or clotting time can be an early warning sign of several different bleeding diseases; some are secondary to other pathology in the body—especially liver disease. Any abnormally long bleeding or clotting time warrants medical consultation. If bleeding time is prolonged but clotting time seems normal, it often indicates thrombocytopenia (a decrease in the number of platelets); with hemophilia-type diseases the bleeding time may be within normal limits while the clotting time is prolonged. These tests, or something similar, should be performed by the doctor or laboratory before any type of surgery.

GLUCOSE

Blood glucose measurements, sometimes called blood sugar measurements, really only measure the amount of one form of sugar, glucose, floating free in the blood at the time of the test. The results primarily show how well the body handles carbohydrate metabolism, and secondarily they show how well all organs related to that metabolism are functioning. No matter what form of sugar (sucrose, or ordinary granulated table sugar; fructose, which is found naturally in fruits; lactose, found in milk products) or other carbohydrates (grains, vegetables) we eat, the body ultimately metabolizes them to glucose (or dextrose, as it is sometimes called). Usually glucose is stored in the liver until it is needed as fuel by the body for many and varied functions: movement of muscles, beating of the heart, breathing, even thinking. If not enough stored glucose is available to fuel these activities, it can then be manufactured from proteins and fat elsewhere in the body. After it is produced, how well glucose is utilized by the body depends a great deal on the hormone insulin, which is secreted by the pancreas—a gland just behind the stomach. The disease known as diabetes is essentially one in which inadequacy or unavailability of insulin prevents proper glucose utilization.

Most often, blood glucose is measured as a single test for screening purposes. It may also be used to note the effects of stress or anxiety on an individual. And single blood glucose measurements are valuable in preventing certain complications that may arise during pregnancy, while dieting, while taking various drugs and subsequent to some forms of poisoning. Should a blood glucose test result suggest an abnormal value, the glucose tolerance test (GTT) is then performed. For this test the individual ingests a measured amount of glucose, usually in liquid form, and the blood glucose levels along with urine **glucose** levels are measured each half-hour for the first two hours and then hourly for the next three hours. This is a more precise evaluation of carbohydrate and glucose metabolism than when a single test is performed. Glucose levels in the blood can also reflect other, non-insulin-related disorders, however, and are influenced by injuries, a variety of hormone-caused diseases, infections and even physical exercise. Many drugs can also cause an elevated blood glucose level, although it is usually temporary. These drugs include:

- Atromid-S—used on some patients with high cholesterol levels
- Birth control pills—oral contraceptives and other estrogens
- Cortisone products—used to treat asthma, arthritis and many skin conditions
- Diuretics
- Nicotinic acid (niacin or vitamin B_3) in large doses over a prolonged period of time
- Tagamet—used to treat stomach ulcers
- Tranquilizers such as Thorazine
- Vitamin A in large doses
- Acetaminophen, the aspirin substitute found in many non-prescription products such as Tylenol, Anacin-3, Pamprin, Sine-Aid and Nyquil.

What Is Usual

If, after a person has gone without any food or drink for two hours or more, the blood glucose level measures anywhere between 60 and 120 mg per 100 ml, this is usually considered normal. Some doctors, however, now consider an occasional level of up to 140 mg per 100 ml as still being within normal limits. After either eating food or drinking a prescribed amount of glucose solution, the blood sugar level should rise no higher than 180 mg per 100 ml and then return to normal limits within two hours. Here again, though, there are doctors who feel that a sudden rise to 240 mg per 100 ml may not necessarily indicate diabetes or other related disease and may be normal for certain individuals. When a glucose tolerance test is performed, the blood sugar level should start out within the accepted normal range, rise markedly in one-half hour and start down at about one hour's time. It should be within normal

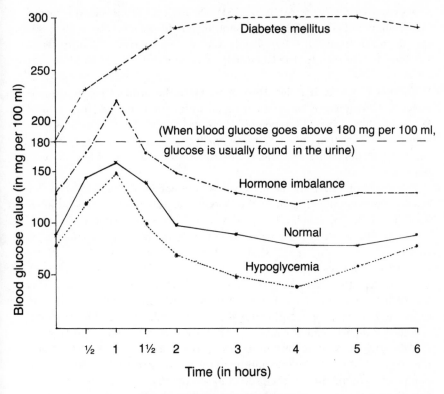

Figure 9. Glucose tolerance test.

limits after two hours, although some people show a drop below their starting figure three or four hours later (Figure 9).

What You Need

A drop of blood (see Blood Tests, **Obtaining a Blood Sample**). The simplest way of measuring the amount of glucose in that drop of blood is to apply it to the tip of a chemically treated plastic test strip, wait one minute, and then wipe it or wash it off and compare the color on the strip to its accompanying color chart, which is calculated to show relative glucose values. One such strip is called Chemstrip bG, and although the numerical values read 20, 40, 80, 120, 180, 240 and 800 mg per 100 ml, it is easy to arrive at values in between those given on the color chart for a reasonably accurate test result—certainly accurate enough for any home testing. Chemstrip bG test strips cost from $10.00 to $15.00 for a package of 25, or about 40 cents per test. Some people cut the test strips in half, lengthwise, using one strip to perform two tests; it reduces the cost by half.

A somewhat similar test strip is VISIDEX; after a drop of blood is placed on the chemically treated tip, it will show blood glucose levels from 20 to 800 mg per ml in from 60 to 90 seconds. Its color comparisons seem easier to distinguish than those of the Chemstrip bG, and it costs $12.00 to $15.00 for 25 strips.

Another test strip is called Dextrostix. Here the drop of blood must be washed off with water, rather than wiped with cotton, and the timing must be absolutely precise. The range of values that can be observed with this test runs from 0 to 250 mg per 100 ml—a smaller range, but allowing a bit more accuracy in comparing the colors. Dextrostix also cost from 40 to 50 cents per test.

The Dextrostix may also be used with a photometer that "reads" the color change electronically and shows the blood sugar value as a specific number on a digital readout display. Such a device, called a Glucometer, while much more expensive, is more precise and eliminates any problem of visual color comparison. The Glucometer shows a blood sugar range from 0 to 399 mg per 100 ml and costs approximately $235.00.

The Dextrostix system also incorporates a synthetic control set that allows a patient to ascertain if the proper procedure is being used and if correct color comparisons are being made. For meter checking, precalibrated solutions are available to allow checks for proper use. Test standardization material, designed to keep a constant check on the quality of the test strips and the accuracy of the technique and instruments, ranges from $1.00 to $5.00 per check. The manufacturer prefers to sell the machines at one of its 350 Self-Testing Centers; contact the Ames Division of Miles Laboratories Inc., P.O. Box 70, Elkhart, Indiana 46515, or call collect: (219) 264–8901 for their location.

The Glucoscan is another company's photometer that gives digital readings from blood sugar test strips. It costs approximately $250.00, but this initial price also includes an automatic finger-pricking device, 200 Monolet lancets, 100 test strips and a control set to assure proper use and accuracy of the machine. Glucoscan test strips cost about 40 cents each. Information about this electronic device can be obtained by calling Lifescan, Inc.: (800) 227–8862.

Both machines are battery-operated, and most health insurance plans will reimburse you for the cost of blood glucose monitors if purchased on the recommendation of your doctor.

Measured amounts of glucose, for glucose tolerance testing, are available as Glucola solution. It costs approximately $1.50 per bottle.

What to Watch Out For
Even before you begin testing, you must be sure that the test strips have been kept absolutely airtight and dry in their containers; air, especially humid air,

leaking into the bottle will deteriorate the test strips and cause false and mis-leading results. If there is any doubt, open a sealed bottle and compare the results of a test with a strip from the old and the new containers. Before testing, be certain that the strip-tip color matches the base standard on the color chart; do not use the strip if the colors do not match. Usually, a deterior-ated test strip will be darker than the standard, or it may show a brownish hue. Most doctors agree that you should not use a test strip from a bottle that has been open more than four months, regardless of the expiration date.

Keep in mind that stress or even anxiety over a seemingly unrelated situa-tion can cause false, elevated blood glucose levels. Most doctors request that their patients make a note of any physical activity, unusual emotional state and dietary intake for the two-hour period prior to testing. Do not test your-self for blood glucose, and particularly for glucose tolerance immediately after any injury, illness or stressful situation; do not perform these tests while di-eting or after any recent weight loss.

Before a glucose tolerance test is performed, it is important to eat a diet containing normal amounts of carbohydrates for several days to a week prior to testing. Many patients tend to cut down drastically on carbohydrates when they plan to have this test, and such dietary alterations can cause false-abnormal results.

Be sure your color vision is normal, since the difference in shades of color between normal and abnormal on some test strips are slight.

What the Test Results Can Mean

A single elevated blood glucose test result (greater than 180 mg per ml) need not be considered significant. Repeated abnormally high test results warrant medical consultation. Only after all the many extraneous factors that can cause a rise in blood glucose levels have been taken into account can a professional investigation be undertaken to ascertain the reason for the abnormally high blood glucose. These extraneous factors include:

• Emotional state
• Food intake for the two or three days prior to testing
• Exercise or other physical exertion for two or three days prior to testing
• Age—blood glucose levels seem to rise normally with age.

In addition to diabetes many other conditions can alter the blood glucose level:

• High blood pressure
• Pregnancy
• Obesity
• Infections

* Heart disease
* Certain cancers
* Various disorders of the pituitary, thyroid, adrenal and pancreas glands
* Recent injuries, especially head trauma or wounds that cause severe bleeding
* Use of certain drugs, especially some of the diuretics.

A lower-than-normal blood glucose level (below 60 mg per 100 ml) can reflect different disorders of the same endocrine glands cited above; it can also reflect inadequate nutrition, prolonged exercise, vomiting for several hours, high fever for several days, liver disease and other metabolic problems, including hypoglycemia. To justify a diagnosis of hypoglycemia, however, blood glucose levels must be lower than 40 mg per 100 ml at least three different times, and such symptoms as sweating, palpitations, weakness and bizarre behavior should be evident along with the low blood glucose levels.

Glucose levels in the urine should correspond to blood glucose levels (see Urine Tests, **Glucose** test).

With a glucose tolerance test, if blood glucose levels are still elevated two hours after drinking the glucose solution, the most common cause is diabetes; as with other abnormally high levels with a single glucose test, however, the cause could be hormonal, injury, infection or emotional. Lower-than-expected glucose values, especially after two hours, can indicate hypoglycemia, pancreatic infection or other causes of excessive insulin production, inadequate production of other body hormones and even anorexia nervosa; they warrant a medical consultation.

Recently, some doctors have employed the glucose tolerance test as a means of detecting certain patients believed to be at a greater risk of having heart disease, especially if the patient has inherited elevated blood lipid levels and is obese.

HEMOGLOBIN

Hemoglobin is an iron-protein substance inside red blood cells that picks up oxygen and gives off carbon dioxide when the blood goes through the lungs. Thus, the amount of oxygen the blood can carry is related to the amount of normal hemoglobin present. There can be many different forms of hemoglobin in blood:

* Carboxyhemoglobin is formed when hemoglobin combines with carbon monoxide, usually as a consequence of smoking (see Breath and Lung Tests, **Carbon Monoxide** test)

- Methemoglobin is formed when hemoglobin combines with food nitrates and many different drugs such as aspirin–like products
- Sulfhemoglobin is formed when hemoglobin combines with certain laxatives and drugs
- Hemoglobin S is associated with sickle cell anemia (see Blood Tests, **Sickle Cell** test)
- Hemoglobin A or A-2 is associated with Mediterranean or Cooley's anemia.

The problem with these abnormal forms of hemoglobin is that they can prevent the normal hemoglobin in the blood from picking up oxygen and thus reduce the body's vital oxygen supply. For self-testing, the measurement of all the many hemoglobins as total hemoglobin is sufficient.

Iron in the diet is the primary source of hemoglobin, and while a minute amount must be replaced regularly, supplements are usually needed after any blood loss, such as from an injury or because of menstruation. Measuring total blood hemoglobin is really only a screening test to indicate anemia, of which there can be a great many causes. And when red blood cells are decreased, either from a condition that prevents their manufacture or from some poison that accelerates their destruction, hemoglobin is often decreased.

What Is Usual
Most men show anywhere from 14 to 16 grams of hemoglobin per 100 ml of blood, while women average from 12 to 15 grams. Young children may show from 11 to 13 grams and still be within normal limits. Sometimes hemoglobin is expressed as a percentage of what is normally expected: Using 15.5 grams as 100 percent, men usually show 90 percent or better (14 grams), while women range at 80 percent or better (12.5 grams).

What You Need
The easiest measure of blood hemoglobin is the standard Tallquist Haemoglobin Scale, where a single drop of blood (see Blood Tests, **Obtaining a Blood Sample**) is placed on a special piece of white blotting paper and then compared with a color scale that accompanies the booklet of blotting papers (Figure 10). The cost averages $2.00 for the color scale and approximately 150 blotting papers. Complete, easy-to-follow directions accompany the booklet. The hemoglobin levels are expressed both in grams per 100 ml and in percentages, with levels for normal hemoglobin, suggestive anemia and actual anemia also indicated. While this version of hemoglobin testing is not precise, it is sufficiently accurate for the usual screening purposes. More precise hemoglobinometers that also use a single drop of blood are available for about $100.00.

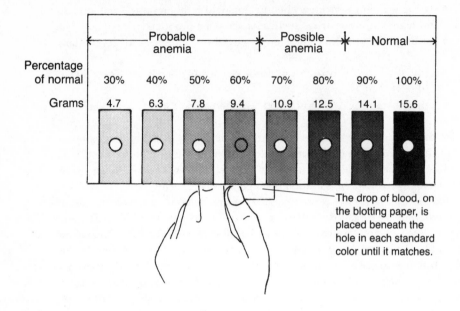

Figure 10. Blood hemoglobin test (for anemia).

What to Watch Out For
Use only one, free-flowing drop of blood on the blotting paper; wipe away any excess with cotton or gauze. Do not wait too long to compare the color of the blood sample with the color chart; it is best to compare the colors within 30 seconds. Use natural light; artificial light can sometimes distort colors. Do not squeeze the fingertip to obtain the blood.

What the Test Results Can Mean
If the color of the spot of blood indicates a lower-than-normal hemoglobin level, especially on more than one testing, it warrants medical consultation. While decreased hemoglobin most often indicates an anemia, the test result does not even hint at the specific cause. Liver disease, thyroid disorders, some inherited conditions, heavy smoking and certain cancers can also lower hemoglobin levels. Some marathon runners develop a mild "sports anemia," which will give a lower-than-normal hemoglobin value, but this usually requires no treatment. It is possible for the test to indicate greater-than-normal values, although exact numbers for values greater than 16 grams are not indicated on the Tallquist color scale. A rare condition such as polycythemia (too many red blood cells), living or working at high altitudes and being dehydrated just prior to testing are the primary causes of an elevated hemoglobin. A persistent higher-than-normal hemoglobin warrants medical consul-

tation. Some doctors believe it could be an early warning sign of an increased risk of a stroke within the brain; some also believe it can be the cause of certain mental problems.

MONONUCLEOSIS

Infectious mononucleosis is also known as dormitory disease, glandular fever, the holiday disease, the kissing disease and students' disease. The origin of the names becomes obvious when one realizes that the condition arises primarily in young people from 10 to 30 years of age, with most cases occurring between 15 and 20 years (although there have been rare cases in 1 year olds and in people over 60), especially in those who room together or who otherwise have repeated close contact. The causative virus can stay in the saliva for more than a year after a person has had the disease. It almost always produces enlarged, tender lymph glands (most often along the side of the neck). And its most common symptoms—fatigue, lethargy, loss of appetite and malaise—are, more often than not, first observed by the young person's parents when their son or daughter comes home from school or college. Other frequent symptoms and signs of the disease include a sore throat (the most common complaint), fever, headache, muscle and stomach pains, swollen eyelids and a rash that can imitate German measles or a drug reaction, or it may look like tiny hemorrhages under the skin. In other words, infectious mononucleosis, in itself an uncomfortable but rarely dangerous disease, can imitate a great many other far more serious conditions and can be very difficult to diagnose. (See Gastrointestinal System Tests, **Mouth and Throat Observations** and Blood Tests, **Streptozyme** test).

The cause of infectious mononucleosis is a herpes-type virus called Epstein-Barr, but because it is difficult to isolate and identify this virus, most tests to help diagnose this disease depend on finding mononucleosis-specific antibodies in the blood. Antibodies are disease-fighting substances formed in the body whenever the body is invaded by microorganisms (bacteria, viruses, etc.); they are usually specific against the infecting germ. The test simply shows whether or not antibodies to the Epstein-Barr virus are present. Antibodies usually appear in the blood of a person with infectious mononucleosis within four or five days after contracting the disease (a day or so before symptoms appear), but they may not be present in a sufficient amount to be detected by testing until two to three weeks later; they may then remain at detectable levels for six months or more.

Several studies have shown that young people with a negative mononucleosis test (no antibodies evident) are much more susceptible to the disease when they leave home for college living; those with a positive test seem to have a degree of immunity.

The test is not perfect. There are other diseases and viruses that can, on occasion, cause a false-positive test. And there are some people who, even though the presence of the disease can be proved by other means, still show a negative test result; a few of these, however, will show a positive test several months after recovering from the disease.

What Is Usual

A negative test is considered normal. An individual with the symptoms and signs that usually accompany infectious mononucleosis has more than a 90 percent chance of showing a positive test reaction if, in fact, the symptoms and signs are from that particular disease. A negative test in the presence of symptoms warrants looking for a different cause of the symptoms.

What You Need

A drop of blood (see Blood Tests, **Obtaining a Blood Sample**) is placed on one of the commercially available slide tests for mononucleosis. They include:

- MONOSTICON-DRI-DOT—a two-minute procedure that costs $16.00 to $22.00 for a 15-test kit; probably the easiest to use
- MONO-TEST (FTB)—the *FTB* stands for fingertip blood—a two-minute test that costs from $22.00 to $25.00 for a 10-test kit.

Each test kit comes with specific instructions, which must be followed explicitly to obtain accurate results.

What to Watch Out For

- If you keep the test material refrigerated, warm it to room temperature before use
- If you are testing someone else's blood, keep in mind that the blood may contain live virus and avoid contact with the blood
- Do not use the test material if it is wet or if, after wetting, it seems cloudy.

What the Test Results Can Mean

Usually the symptoms and signs of infectious mononucleosis are such that they warrant medical attention. If, however, they seem mild or inconsequential, a mononucleosis test might help point to a diagnosis. If the test is positive, no matter how slight the symptoms, a medical consultation is warranted.

If the test is negative but symptoms are present, the test should be repeated in one week. If the symptoms become annoying or persist, a medical consultation is warranted no matter what the test result; infectious mononucleosis can have drastic, although rare, complications. A negative test without symptoms or signs of any illness usually indicates susceptibility to the disease and can offer useful information should a mysterious illness occur at a later date.

RHEUMATOID FACTOR (Arthritis)

The symptoms of arthritis—pain and stiffness in the joints, usually but not always accompanied by swelling, redness and warmth of the afflicted joints—can come from many different diseases. When the joint stiffness is worse after inactivity, especially first thing in the morning, and when there are repeated bouts of fever, along with weight loss and generalized weakness, the most likely diagnosis is rheumatoid arthritis, a prolonged inflammatory-response disease that affects the entire body. It usually occurs between 20 and 60 years of age and more than twice as often in women as in men. Although the specific cause is still unknown (some doctors feel it comes from a virus, while others blame genetics, diet and even emotional stress), at least three out of four people with rheumatoid arthritis produce special antibodies called rheumatoid factor, which can be tested for, and detected, in the blood. Antibodies are manufactured in response to, and to help combat, infections and many other disease antigens (the disease-provoking substances). Unfortunately, other nonarthritic conditions can also cause a rheumatoid factor reaction—especially liver, lung and heart problems; syphilis; and certain worm (parasite) infestations. The test is performed primarily on patients with arthritis, or on those with unexplained eye or skin conditions, to help in the confirmation of a diagnosis and to select proper treatment. Rheumatoid factor usually does not appear in the blood until months after the disease begins, and it can persist for several years. A negative test does not rule out a diagnosis of rheumatoid arthritis, but it can help distinguish between other rheumatoid conditions that damage joints; muscles; collagen, or connective tissue; and various bodily organs.

What Is Usual
There should be no evidence of rheumatoid factor in the blood (a negative test). If rheumatoid arthritis has been diagnosed, however, about 97 percent of those correctly diagnosed will show a positive test.

What You Need
A drop of blood (see Blood Tests, **Obtaining a Blood Sample**) is placed on a designated dot on a paper slide that is part of a RHEUMANOSTICAN DRI-DOT kit, which costs from $18.00 to $20.00 for 25 test kits; two large test tubes, which cost from 50 cents to $1.00 each; and some calibrated capillary tubes, which cost $2.00 per 100.

What to Watch Out For
• This test kit comes with positive and negative control samples; when using the kit for the first time, test yourself with the controls to be sure you are performing the test properly

• Do not use a test kit if the seal or envelope has been broken; if there is only one dot on the slide (there should be two—one peach-colored and one clear); if the slide appears to be moist
• Use a sweep-second hand or digital display seconds clock or watch, or a stopwatch, to time the one minute that the test takes.

What the Test Results Can Mean
This test is a prime example of the fact that any medical test result alone—be it positive or negative, within normal numerical limits or higher or lower than what is usually found in ostensibly normal, healthy people—is not conclusive proof of the presence or absence of a suspected disease or condition. A positive rheumatoid factor test, even if accompanied by the usual symptoms and signs of rheumatoid arthritis, is but one peg on which to hang a proper diagnosis. It must be kept in mind, however, that the test is not definitive and that a positive reaction can also occur with:

• Other forms of arthritis-mimicking conditions, such as gout, ankylosing spondylitis (stiffening of the spine, primarily), psoriasis, colitis, gonorrhea and other joint infections.
• Diseases of collagen (which is the connective tissue under the skin, around organs, bones, muscles and other structures that helps hold everything together), such as systemic lupus erythematosus and scleroderma.
• Generalized infections, such as tuberculosis, leprosy, syphilis and endocarditis (infection of the lining of the heart).

And a positive reaction has been known to occur in evidently healthy people with no signs of an arthritic involvement. A positive test warrants medical consultation.

A negative test simply means that rheumatoid factor antibodies are not present or are present in such minute amounts as to be undetectable. It would seem that symptoms providing sufficient provocation to perform this test would warrant medical consultation, even if the test result is negative.

SICKLE CELL

Sickle cells are red blood cells that carry a misshapen molecule of hemoglobin called hemoglobin S (see Blood Tests, **Hemoglobin** test), which, in turn, causes these cells to assume a "sickle" shape (somewhat like the curved blade used for farming) instead of the usual doughnut shape of normal red blood cells. Because of their elongated shape, sickle cells cannot pass through tiny arteries and capillaries and can cause small clots (thromboses), which prevent adequate blood from reaching distant tissues. Sickle cells are also much more fragile than normal red blood cells and tend to break easily, causing anemia. These changes occur more frequently when there are lower-than-normal amounts of oxygen, such as when flying, after injuries or during surgery, and can precipitate a critical, sometimes fatal condition.

There are two distinct aspects of sickle cell problems: sickle cell anemia, in which the individual inherits more than one sickle cell-causing gene and actually contracts the disease, and sickle cell trait (sickling trait), in which only one sickle cell-causing gene is inherited and the individual does not show any signs of the disease. If, by chance, two people with sickle cell trait mate, they can pass the disease on to their offspring.

The disease shows itself through severe episodes of pain, especially in the abdomen and bones when these organs are deprived of blood; weakness and jaundice from the anemia; as well as nerve and muscle disorders when the brain is afflicted. Those with only the trait rarely show any symptoms unless exposed to extremes of diminished oxygen. Both, however, may at times show physical signs (blood in the urine, swelling of the hands and feet, and pain imitating appendicitis or gallstones) that can confuse doctors and cause them to suspect some disease other than sickle cell anemia unless the sickle cells are known to be present. Thus, the importance of screening for sickle cell hemoglobin.

Although the disease and the trait are found primarily in blacks (1 out of every 400 inherits the disease; 1 out of every 10 inherits the trait), they are also found in Caucasians of Mediterranean or Middle Eastern origin. And if someone with sickle cells needs surgery, the anesthetist must know about the condition in order to supply the patient with adequate oxygen.

What Is Usual
No evidence of hemoglobin S should be detected in the blood.

What You Need
A Sickledex Tube Test kit, which costs from $22.00 to $28.00 for a package of 12 test kits. A drop or two of blood (see Blood Tests, **Obtaining a Blood Sample**) is placed in the tube.

What to Watch Out For
Do not test infants younger than 3 months of age. If hemoglobin S is present but in low levels in infants the test could show a false-negative result; it should be repeated a few months later.

What the Test Results Can Mean
Because the test does not distinguish between sickle cell disease and sickle cell trait, any positive test warrants immediate medical attention. If anemia exists,

or if symptoms similar to sickle cell disease occur, a medical consultation is warranted, even in the face of a negative test.

STREPTOZYME (Streptococcus Infections)

Streptococci bacteria are the most common cause of a sore throat or pharyngitis (an inflammation of the pharynx, or the area in back of the throat behind the tongue). Streptococci can also cause severe skin infections, ear infections, meningitis, blood poisoning and scarlet fever. Although the majority of streptococcus infections can be treated with the proper antibiotics, a missed diagnosis, a delay in treatment, application of inadequate or improper antibiotics, or use of the antibiotic for an insufficient time (10 days is the minimum) can allow dangerous secondary effects to develop:

- Rheumatic fever, which can destroy the valves of the heart
- Nephritis, a severe, sometimes fatal kidney disease that can last for years
- Erysipelas, a skin condition (especially of the cheeks) that is particularly dangerous in very young or very old people.

As with many diseases, the streptococci, which are disease-provoking antigens, cause the body to produce antibodies to that specific bacteria, and it is the presence of such antibodies that is the basis for the streptococcal infection test. Once these antibodies are found to be present—especially within a week or two following a sore throat, earache or skin infection—appropriate measures can be undertaken to avoid the potentially lethal consequences of a streptococcus infection. As only one example, the American Heart Association still claims that more than 10,000 people will die from rheumatic fever each year.

A sore throat can come from many other illnesses (see Gastrointestinal System Tests, **Mouth and Throat Observation** and Blood Tests, **Mononucleosis** test), just as an earache may not necessarily be caused by bacteria (see Ear Observations and Hearing Tests, **Ear Canal and Eardrum Observations**).

What Is Usual
While most people have been exposed to streptococcus at one time or another, it is still unusual to show a positive result with this test unless there has been a recent exposure to a streptococcus infection.

What You Need
- A STREPTOZYME two-minute slide test kit, which costs from $20.00 to $25.00 for 15 test kits

- Normal (isotonic) saline (contains the same amount of salt as body fluids); a one-ounce bottle costs 60 to 75 cents, while an eight-ounce bottle costs from $5.00 to $6.00; but you need only 2.5 ml, or less than one-tenth of an ounce, for each test
- A drop of blood (see Blood Tests, **Obtaining a Blood Sample**) is placed on the slide and diluted with the normal saline according to the test kit's directions
- A 3 to 5 ml capacity syringe and needle to measure out the saline; they cost from 15 to 25 cents each
- A test tube, which costs from 50 cents to $1.00
- A watch for timing.

What to Watch Out For
Each test kit comes with a control specimen, which should show a positive reaction; first perform the test with this control to assure yourself that your procedure is correct. As another check, perform the test with saline; it should show a negative reaction. Follow the instructions precisely. Be sure the test tube and syringe are clean and dry; any cleaning material left on the surface can give a false result.

If you are already taking antibiotics or using cortisone-type drugs, do not count on the test results; these drugs can cause a false-negative test.

What the Test Results Can Mean
A positive test indicates more than the usual amount of streptococci antibodies are present and, if associated with any symptoms or signs of illness, especially a sore throat, warrants immediate medical attention. A positive test, even where no symptoms are evident, still warrants a medical consultation. A negative result could mean the test was performed too early in the course of the illness and should be repeated in a day or two. Even a negative test, in the presence of possible streptococci-caused symptoms such as fever, sore throat or skin infection, warrants medical consultation.

Although this test is only a screening device and its results must be confirmed by more specific tests, it could allow someone with a previously unidentified streptococcus infection to seek proper medical help early enough to prevent more serious illness.

UREA NITROGEN (Blood Urea Nitrogen, BUN)

Urea is produced in the liver and is the main nitrogen-containing end product of protein metabolism. Normally, there is very little urea in blood, and what is present is usually eliminated into the urine by the kidneys. A diet high in protein can cause a temporary increase in blood urea nitrogen (BUN), as can excessive exercise with profuse perspiration and other activities that cause dehydration or starvation, such as vomiting and/or diarrhea. A low-protein diet can decrease BUN values. And the use of a great many drugs can alter BUN levels:

- Antibiotics, such as Chloromycetin and streptomycin
- Diuretic drugs
- Blood pressure medications, such as methyldopa
- Salicylates, such as aspirin and related products
- Sedatives, such as chloral hydrate
- Steroid hormones, such as cortisone products.

Although the BUN is primarily an indicator of kidney function, it can be altered by so many other non-kidney-related conditions that it should be considered only as a rough screening test for kidney disease and as an early warning signal for other latent body pathology.

What Is Usual
Most people show a BUN of from 10 to 20 mg per 100 ml of blood. Repeated values within this range are reasonably indicative of normal kidney function. It is possible to have a value less than 10 mg per 100 ml following a low-protein diet and during pregnancy.

What You Need
A drop of blood (see Blood Tests, **Obtaining a Blood Sample**) and an AZO-STIX (a plastic strip with a chemically treated tip, similar to those used in blood glucose and urine testing), which costs from $14.00 to $18.00 for a package of 25. Incidentally, the prefix *azo* refers to nitrogen, and azotemia means too much urea nitrogen in the blood.

What to Watch Out For
- Do not use the AZOSTIX if the chemically treated tip has a yellowish color
- Do not use an AZOSTIX that has been in a bottle more than 60 days after opening, no matter what the expiration date given
- Do not use a small drop of blood; a large drop is required
- Use a sweep-second hand or digital display clock or watch, or a stop-watch, for this test; exact timing of one minute is extremely important
- Color distinction is critical; be sure you have normal color vision
- Be sure to take any drugs you are using into consideration; consult your doctor or pharmacist to see if your medicines will interfere with this test.

What the Test Results Can Mean

Any test result that is between 15 and 20 mg per 100 ml should be repeated the next day. If still close to 20 mg per 100 ml, a medical consultation is warranted. A test value greater than 20 mg per 100 ml is abnormal, and even if the cause can be explained by diet, physical activity or drug use, it warrants medical attention. There are other tests a doctor can perform to ascertain whether the high BUN is from a disease. Most often, an increase in BUN is an indication of kidney trouble; it may be from an acute infection, from repeated damage due to chronic infection or from a tumor. Any other condition that causes less blood to flow through the kidneys, such as heart failure, bleeding, shock and even extreme stress, can cause an elevated BUN. Other things that can increase the BUN include: heavy-metal poisoning; thyroid disease; diabetes; gout; many different hormone disorders; infections elsewhere in the body, such as pneumonia and pancreatitis or simply a high fever; and any blockage of the urinary tract, such as from a kidney stone, bladder infection or enlarged prostate (see Urine Tests, **Urine Flow Rate** and **Nitrite** tests). Again, a BUN greater than 20 mg per 100 ml warrants immediate medical attention.

On occasion, the BUN can be lowered by liver disease, from certain drugs, a condition called amyloidosis (an accumulation of a starchlike material throughout the body) and nephrosis (a degenerative disease of the kidneys that causes water retention, or edema). A persistent decreased BUN warrants medical consultation.

BREATH AND LUNG TESTS

PULMONARY FUNCTION MEASUREMENTS

Measurement of dynamic lung functions—how much air the lungs can hold and how well that air can be expelled—provides valuable clues to the cause of breathing problems. When performed on a regular basis, these tests can also offer early warning signals of newly developing or latent lung disease. In addition, lung-air evaluations are helpful in selecting the most effective treatment as well as in following the progress of therapy. Dynamic lung measurements are only a small part of overall pulmonary function testing, which usually includes an additional half-dozen laboratory-controlled breathing tests as well as gas diffusion tests, which show the effectiveness of the transfer of oxygen from the lungs to the blood and of carbon dioxide from the blood back to the lungs.

For home testing, the simple "match test," the forced expiratory time test, and two or three breathing tests using a spirometer (an instrument that records the exact amount of air passing through it and, at times, the rate of air passage during a specific time), or one test using a peak flow meter can offer information concerning the possible presence of lung problems.

There are two basic categories of lung pathology: the obstructive type and the restrictive type (Figure 11). The obstructive type is the most common cause of shortness of breath (dyspnea). It can come from:

- Asthma, either brought on by an allergy, repeated lung infections or by exercise
- Bronchiectasis, where the bronchi lose their ability to contract and thus can no longer help expel mucous; this usually follows prolonged, severe lung infections
- Chronic bronchitis, as an active, long-standing infection
- Cystic fibrosis, where excessive mucous production blocks air movement within the bronchi (See Breath and Lung tests; **Skin Saltiness**)
- Emphysema, where the lung's elasticity is insufficient to expel air easily
- Drugs, particularly those used to treat heart disease, glaucoma and joint pains.

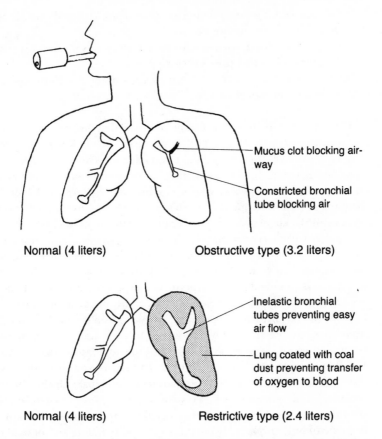

Mucus clot blocking air-way

Constricted bronchial tube blocking air

Normal (4 liters)   Obstructive type (3.2 liters)

Inelastic bronchial tubes preventing easy air flow

Lung coated with coal dust preventing transfer of oxygen to blood

Normal (4 liters)   Restrictive type (2.4 liters)

Figure 11. Measuring the lungs' forced vital capacity using a Windmill-type spirometer.

With the restrictive type of lung disease, the lungs are unable to fill with air, or if air does enter the lungs, the normal free and easy passage of oxygen to the blood is impaired. Restrictive lung problems can come from:

- An injury to, or deformity of, the ribs or the chest wall; any condition that causes severe pain when trying to take a deep breath can also result in a similar problem
- Pulmonary fibrosis, where normal lung tissue is replaced by scarlike tissue; this can come from an old infection or from inhaling irritating particles, such as asbestos, coal dust, cotton dust, fungi and a host of industrial chemicals
- Certain nerve or muscle diseases that affect the diaphragm or rib cage, such as myasthenia gravis or muscular dystrophy

• Any loss of lung tissue; either from its being replaced by a growing tumor or as a consequence of surgery
• Pulmonary edema, where fluids fill the air spaces within or surrounding the lungs, such as happens with pleurisy
• Pregnancy, if the enlarged uterus presses up on the diaphragm; this, of course, is only temporary.

The six basic lung tests that can be performed at home include:

The match test. The "match test" is performed by holding a lighted paper match six inches from the open mouth, taking in as deep a breath as possible and then exhaling the air as forcibly as possible in order to blow out the match (you must not pucker your lips to increase the force of the air flow, but keep the mouth wide open). The ability to perform this test successfully usually means the chances of an existing lung problem are remote.

The forced expiratory time test (FET). Another "open-mouth" test requires a watch with a second hand or digital display second measurements (a stopwatch is more accurate but not required). In the "match test" the goal was to test the *force* of exhaled air; in the forced expiratory time test, the goal is to measure the *time* it takes to exhale all the air the lungs can hold. With a watch in front of you, breathe in as deeply as you possibly can. With your mouth wide open, exhale as forcibly and as fast as you can and count the seconds from the instant you start to exhale until the very last bit of air is expelled. You should repeat this test several times and record your best (shortest) time. Most people without any lung impairment can exhale all their lung air in from two to six seconds. If it takes you more than five seconds to exhale all your lung air, it could be a warning signal of either an obstructive or restrictive type of lung problem. It warrants spirometry testing and/or medical consultation.

The following three tests require the use of a spirometer:

forced vital capacity test (FVC). Forced vital capacity (FVC) measures just how *much* air the lungs can forcibly exhale after taking in as large a breath as possible (Figure 12). This is really the simplest recordable standardized indication of the lungs' condition.

forced expiratory volume in one second test (FEV$_1$). This test is usually performed at the same time as the forced vital capacity; it measures the exact amount of air being blown out during the first second of the FVC test (Figure 12). The FVC and the FEV$_1$ tests together can sometimes discriminate between an obstructive and a restrictive type of lung condition.

maximal voluntary ventilation test (MVV). This test offers a record of the greatest amount of air a person can forcibly breathe in and out in one minute's time (the test is usually conducted for 12 to 15 seconds and the amount multiplied by either 5 or 4). Formerly called maximum breathing capacity, this test is a

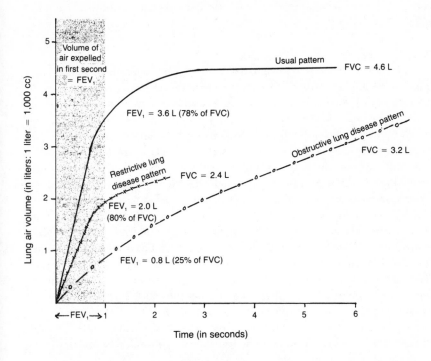

Figure 12. Typical patterns of forced vital capacity (FVC) and forced expiratory volume in one second (FEV₁) tests.

relative indication of the lungs' physical fitness, since it also takes into account the muscles that help you breathe and how well you coordinate all breathing-related activities.

peak expiratory flow rate test (PEFR). This test measures the maximal expiratory flow rate during a forcible exhalation after taking in as much air as the lungs can hold. For this test, it is not necessary to exhale every bit of air. It requires a peak flow meter. (While not as accurate as the spirometer, this particular device is being recommended more and more by doctors because of its low cost, simplicity of use and minimal maintenance.) The PEFR test is a reasonable reflection of the amount of air exhaled in approximately the first second when compared to the FEV_1; another difference is that the exhaled air is translated into a rate-time result—some meters report it in liters per minute (L/min.), others in liters per second (L/sec.). The PEFR test (sometimes called the Peak Flow Rate) is most commonly used by asthmatic patients at home to assist the doctor in monitoring their condition, evaluating drug effectiveness and identifying early warning signs to prevent impending severe attacks. For nonasthmatics it can offer an indication of obstructive lung disease.

What Is Usual

Dynamic lung functions are evaluated, using a spirometer, by measuring the quantity of air exhaled in liters (L) or cubic centimeters (cc). (One liter is equivalent to 1,000 cubic centimeters and is slightly more than a quart.)

The forced vital capacity (FVC) test values depend on one's age, height and sex. The larger (usually taller) a person is, the larger the lung capacity is expected to be. The younger a person is, the more elastic the lung tissues and chest muscles, and this should result in an ability to exhale air from the lungs much more forcibly. And since men usually have larger chest wall dimensions along with stronger chest muscles, they are expected to have a greater forced vital capacity than women. All spirometers come with a chart or table that shows expected test values for different ages, heights and sex. Two examples: A man 5½ feet tall, from 25 to 55 years of age, should have an FVC of at least four liters (4000 cc); a woman five feet tall, from 15 to 55 years of age, should have an FVC of at least three liters (3,000 cc). But such figures are not absolute; a deviation of 20 percent either way from the values shown on the chart or table supplied with the spirometer is still considered within normal limits, and many doctors do not consider a 25 percent deviation abnormal. Thus, if the expected value is supposed to be four liters, any result from three to five liters can also be normal.

The forced expiratory volume in one second (FEV₁) test is really a refinement of the forced vital capacity test. Usually, a person without a lung problem will forcibly breathe out from 75 percent to 80 percent of the total forced vital capacity within the first second of exhalation. If, for example, the forced vital capacity was four liters, then at least three liters should have been expelled within the first second of exhalation.

The maximal voluntary ventilation (MVV) test, measuring the amount of air going in and out of the lungs during a 12 or 15 second period of time (as opposed to a single forced exhalation) while breathing as hard and as fast as possible is most often expressed as liters per minute (L/min.) After 12 or 15 seconds the total amount of recorded air volume is multiplied by five or four, and it should be at least 15 to 20 times the forced vital capacity volume. Someone with a forced vital capacity of four liters should have a maximal voluntary ventilation rate of at least 60 L/min. and closer to 80 L/min. A well-trained athlete can have an MVV of more than 30 times the FVC.

The peak expiratory flow rate test also takes an individual's age, height and sex into consideration (as does the FEV). Each test instrument, no matter of what design, is accompanied by "predicted normal values" expressed in L/min. or L/sec. Many doctors consider a test result within 75 percent to 80 percent of the usual flow rate, as shown on the tables, to be within normal limits. Patients with asthma or other lung conditions usually establish their own baseline in consultation with their doctors so as to be aware of significant changes. In general, a man 5½ feet tall, from 25 to 55 years of age, will show a PEFR of from 500 to 600 L/min. (6 to 9 L/sec.). A woman five feet tall, from 15 to 55 years of age, will average from 400 to 500 L/min. (5 to 8 L/sec.).

What You Need
A spirometer is required. These instruments come in many shapes and sizes—all easily hand-held. The simplest spirometers will only measure forced vital capacity (FVC) and maximal voluntary ventilation (MVV). The Propper-style compact spirometer is reportedly the most accurate of all the small-sized breath measuring devices; it uses a dial showing divisions in tenths of a liter and costs from $100.00 to $140.00. A very accurate spirometer that in addition to measuring FVC and MVV also measures the forced expiratory flow in one second (FEV_1) is the Windmill (battery-operated), which shows air volume in digital display figures and costs $85.00. Other similar home-use devices can cost up to $300.00.

There are many different kinds of peak flow meters available, but keep in mind that these instruments measure PEFR only. To name a few:

- The Organon peak flow meter, which costs $10.00 to $15.00
- The Sears Roebuck Lung Power Monitor, which costs $17.00
- The Vitalograph Pulmonary Monitor, which costs $18.00
- The Armstrong Mini-Wright peak flow meter, which costs $60.00
- The Armstrong Professional peak flow meter, which costs $445.00.

What to Watch Out For
Be sure your spirometer is working properly. Although all hand-held spirometers are sufficiently accurate for home testing, they do tend to become inaccurate after a period of time. One way is to check it out with your doctor's office machine. Another way is to have someone whose FVC is known and normal help calibrate your spirometer.

Avoid even the slightest breathing through the nose while testing. If this seems difficult, apply a nose clip or pinch the tip of your nose. Be sure your lips are sealed tightly around the mouthpiece while exhaling.

It really does not matter whether you sit or stand when performing spirometry, but you should assume a position that will allow you to take in the largest possible breath and blow it out as forcibly and continuously as you can until every bit of air is exhaled.

Do not accept only one test result, or even the first few; rest and repeat the tests until two or more results are almost identical and then record the highest value.

What the Test Results Can Mean

The most common indication of a possible chest problem is a reduced forced vital capacity (FVC) test. If your test result is 70 percent of what would be expected for your age, height and sex, or less, it could mean either an obstructive or a restrictive lung condition. If less than normally expected FVC values are observed on three or more occasions, a medical consultation is warranted.

If the forced expiratory volume in one second (FEV_1) is less than 75 percent of your FVC, a lung problem is more apt to be of the obstructive type. A reduced maximum voluntary ventilation (MVV) is also an indication of an obstructive type of lung condition, and medical consultation is warranted.

If the forced vital capacity is reduced, but the forced expiratory volume in one second and the maximal voluntary ventilation tests are near normal, it may be a sign of a restrictive type of lung problem, and a medical consultation is warranted.

A supplementary procedure that tends to point to an obstructive-type problem, and one that also helps indicate how treatable that problem can be, is the *bronchodilator inhalation challenge test*. After establishing your baseline values for FVC and FEV_1, you inhale from a bronchodilator dispenser containing epinephrine (adrenalin); Bronkaid Mist and Primatine Mist are two such products. With lung problems due to allergy, the epinephrine will usually increase the FVC within 15 minutes. Although these drugs are sold without a prescription, do not use one of these inhalers until you first discuss it with your doctor; they can cause a rapid heartbeat, elevate the blood pressure and produce nervousness. Many doctors advise their patients who have asthma to obtain a spirometer or peak flow meter and keep a record of their breathing difficulties—such as when they occur and what seems to provoke them—and the measurable amount of relief obtained with the use of various medicines.

Another observation that can indicate lung problems is a large difference between FVC and FEV_1 measurements from day to day. People with obstructive types of lung disease tend to show such variations which warrant a medical consultation.

And recent research indicates that a reduced forced vital capacity test, even in the absence of any lung problems, seems to be a warning sign of impending heart failure.

A decreased peak expiratory flow rate (PEFR) of less than 80 percent below predicted values accompanying the peak flow meter warrants medical consultation. While it most often indicates an airway obstruction due to asthma, it is also a reasonable single, simple, evaluation of lung function. It can be very valuable in uncovering asthma without wheezing and breathing difficulties due to exercise or exertion. For someone with known asthma, regular testing with a peak flow meter can offer an early warning signal of an impending asthmatic attack and can help ward off that attack.

Peak flow meters have proved of value to those trying to stop smoking. The obvious objective improvement in lung function in ex-smokers along with the evident loss of lung power should smoking begin again offers a real incentive to abstain from smoking.

The most recent medical research has associated impotence with the obstructive type of lung disease; it seems that sexual dysfunction decreases in direct proportion to the degree that lung function tests values are reduced (see Genitourinary System Tests: **Nocturnal Penile Tumescence Screening**). Evidence of impotence accompanied by any decrease in lung function certainly warrants a medical consultation.

If any dynamic lung function test shows repeated deviation from what is expected, medical consultation is warranted.

BREATH ALCOHOL

While testing for the body's alcohol content—whether through breath, blood or urine—is most often related to the legal question of drunken driving, breath alcohol levels can be of even greater value if measured *prior* to driving after drinking. There are many people who actually test themselves, at home, with known amounts of beer, liquors and wine to learn just how much they can consume before reaching the legal level of "being under the influence." Others test their guests at the end of a party (some states make a host responsible for any damages by a drunken guest). People vary tremendously in how much alcohol it takes to impair their mental and physical abilities; and different states have widely varying limits of blood alcohol levels that constitute violation of the law. Knowing how much alcohol it takes for *you* to reach impairment (some people cannot drive a car safely after only one or two drinks) can prevent many alcohol-caused diseases and could save lives.

Scientific studies have shown that proper testing of breath alcohol is as accurate as, and is equivalent to, direct blood measurements. Breath alcohol tests measure the body's content of ethyl alcohol or ethanol, the kind of alcohol used for consumption. This is in contrast to isopropyl alcohol or propanol, commonly used as rubbing alcohol, antifreeze or as a solvent; and methyl alcohol, also known as methanol or wood alcohol, which is used in plastics manufacturing and for cleaning purposes. Small amounts of the latter two alcohols can be fatal.

An ounce of average 86 proof liquor (proof is twice the percentage of alcohol in the beverage) contains about the same amount of alcohol (10 grams, 10,000 mg or 1/3 of an ounce) as do eight ounces of beer or four ounces of wine. After alcohol is consumed, it reaches its peak blood level in about half an hour. Three ounces of an average liquor will usually produce some symptoms of intoxication and can cause a blood alcohol level measurement of over 0.05 percent (in a few states, sufficient for a person to be considered legally drunk). Ten ounces of the same proof alcohol will usually produce stupor or coma; blood alcohol measurements reflect this state with a level of 0.4 percent. Twelve ounces of ethyl alcohol at one time have caused death. It takes from two to three hours to eliminate each ounce of alcohol from the body.

Most states consider 0.10 percent body alcohol measurements, whether by blood or breath, as evidence of intoxication (in England 0.08 percent is the legal limit); some states, however, insist on a measurement of 0.15 percent before issuing a citation. A level of 0.10 percent means that there are 100 mg of pure alcohol in every 3⅓ ounces of blood; as a comparison, it takes only one-thousandth as much (0.1 mg) Dilantin (a drug used to treat epilepsy) in the blood to be effective enough to prevent convulsions.

What Is Usual
Obviously, no measurable amount of alcohol in the body would be normal. Legally, a breath alcohol level of less than 0.05 percent is rarely considered intoxication.

What You Need
A portable, battery-operated breath alcohol meter (the AlcoCheck is one brand name, ATC-1 is another), which can cost anywhere from $60.00 to $90.00. After breathing into the device, it may signal alcohol content by colored lights; green means less than 0.05 percent; yellow means from 0.05 percent to 0.10 percent; red means more than 0.10 percent. Other alcohol breath test meters show the exact alcohol content on a dial gauge or in digital display numbers. These instruments may be used repeatedly. A one-time disposable test is the National Drager AlcoTest, comprised of a breathing bag and a glass alcohol-indication tube; these cost $33.00 for a 10-test package.

What to Watch Out For
Do not attempt to measure breath alcohol for at least 15 minutes after your last drink; during that time there is enough alcohol in your mouth and saliva to cause a false result. Do not attempt to test if you just rinsed your mouth with mouthwash; many contain alcohol and will cause false results. If you are diabetic, you can have a falsely elevated breath (blood) alcohol test if you are also forming ketones in your body (see Urine Tests, **Ketones**). Do not smoke just prior to taking the test; tobacco smoke can, at times, distort some color tests. Be sure the device is operating properly. In 1982 more than 1,000 Breathalyzer machines (used primarily by police departments) were found to be defective, causing erroneous breath alcohol readings.

What the Test Results Can Mean
Testing could, of course, help save hundreds of dollars, prevent the loss of your driver's license, keep you out of jail and avoid humiliation—not to men-

tion the lives that might be saved. Keep in mind, however, that the breath alcohol test does not indicate how much alcohol was imbibed or whether alcoholism exists, nor does it necessarily indicate your degree of impairment; it simply reflects the blood alcohol level at the time the test was performed. It cannot tell if alcohol was used within 30 minutes prior to the test, which could cause a higher blood level a short while later. Most of all, the test can help to keep social drinking within a reasonably safe level and could be a means to prevent alcoholism (see Brain and Nervous System Tests, **Alcoholism** test).

BREATH CARBON MONOXIDE

When carbon monoxide is mentioned, most people think primarily of an automobile's exhaust fumes and their deadly effects. Carbon monoxide is, in fact, a colorless, odorless, tasteless gas—only one small fraction of exhaust gases—which, when inhaled, can cause a multitude of symptoms: dizziness, dyspnea (shortness of breath), fainting, giddiness, headache, impaired judgment, memory loss, muscle paralysis, ringing in the ears, unconsciousness, vomiting and ultimately death; it can worsen all sorts of existing heart disease. In addition, exposure to carbon monoxide has been shown to decrease estrogen (female hormone) production and bring on an earlier than normal menopause. The diminished amount of estrogens is also believed to increase the risk of osteoporosis (weakened bone structure) and spinal vertebrae fractures. In men, increased carbon monoxide in the blood decreases testosterone (male hormone) production and can be a cause of impotence (see Genitourinary System Tests, **Nocturnal Penile Tumescence Screening**).

Carbon monoxide acts by replacing normal oxygen-carrying hemoglobin in the blood with carboxyhemoglobin, a compound that prevents life-supporting oxygen from reaching the brain and nerves as well as all the other body organs. One gram of carboxyhemoglobin can replace 200 grams of normal hemoglobin. If not fatal, exposure to small amounts at repeated intervals can cause permanent nerve and muscle damage. Carbon *mon*oxide (its symbol is CO as opposed to CO_2, the symbol for carbon *di*oxide, the harmless bubbles in soft drinks) can come from many sources:

- Defective or improperly ventilated heaters and furnaces—even home fireplaces
- Industrial plants that manufacture organic chemicals
- Refineries where coke is burned
- Any situation involving burning where the process of combustion is incomplete
- Service garages and those attached to homes
- Automobile tunnels

• Buildings that generate electric power from gasoline-run engines
• Gasoline powered lawn mowers
• Charcoal barbecue fires with inadequate ventilation
• Smoking—tobacco, marijuana or any other plant.

While most blood tests for carbon monoxide are complicated laboratory procedures, it is fairly simple to detect and measure the amount of carboxyhemoglobin in the blood by testing for the amount of carbon monoxide in the breath. It usually requires at least a 50 percent concentration of carboxyhemoglobin to cause fainting or unconsciousness, but more than 2 percent can cause mental impairment and more than 60 percent can be fatal. It takes no more than 10 percent to cause headache and shortness of breath; over 30 percent can make you dizzy, impair your judgment, impair your vision and make you extremely agitated.

Smoking when pregnant can cause a marked decrease in oxygen to the brain and body of the fetus; proportionately much more than to the expectant mother. And the loss of oxygen to the baby persists for hours after the mother stops smoking.

What Is Usual
A recent government survey of blood carboxyhemoglobin levels showed that, as a possible result of air pollution, just about everyone—even children under 3 years of age—shows some exposure to carbon monoxide (on the average of 1 percent to 2 percent). Those who smoke cigarettes, cigars or pipes, however, had more than four times that level of blood carboxyhemoglobin—some showing more than 10 percent. Thus, the government reports that the greatest source of carbon monoxide poisoning is smoking; only one pack of cigarettes a day can cause persistent carboxyhemoglobin levels of 10 percent.

What You Need
Carbon monoxide breath testing requires a Draegar CO breath test kit that includes a special glass tube into which you instill your exhaled air. Although the cost of each test comes to $6.40, there is an initial cost of $140.00 for a special Bellows Pump (necessary for standardization of the amount of breath to be measured). Most laboratories charge at least $30.00 for a single blood test. Obviously, the cost must be taken into consideration, but it can be considered relatively inexpensive if it justifies the stopping of smoking and subsequently relieves previously unexplained symptoms. It can be of even greater value if it uncovers home or work areas that contain dangerous levels of the gas, thus preventing future damage or revealing the cause of one or more physical or emotional problems. No technical training is needed to perform the test.

CARBON MONOXIDE MONITORING

To check for areas in your home, garage, automobile or work environment that might contain carbon monoxide, you can purchase CO Leak-Tec area contamination monitors; these small detectors can be mounted on walls (they have adhesive backs) or around pipes and reveal CO through a color change. There are also Leak-Tec personal protection badges that can be worn while in suspected areas. They are available from American Gas & Chemical Company, Northvale, NJ 07647 and cost $35.00 for a package of 12 tests (minimum order) that includes the test button and holder; replacement test buttons cost $20.00 per dozen. These detectors will also reveal the amount of carbon monoxide in a room while smoking. Once a test button turns color to show carbon monoxide, it must be replaced.

A permanent carbon monoxide detector-alert that sounds an alarm when dangerous amounts of CO are present is available from Hammacher Schlemmer in New York City or by mail for $70.00.

What to Watch Out For
Do not perform the breath test in an environment where carbon monoxide might exist, such as at one's place of work, a room at home that is suspect or even a room where someone is, or has recently been, smoking. It could cause false-elevated breath values.

What the Test Results Can Mean
Although the presence of more than 5 percent carboxyhemoglobin is not absolute proof that carbon monoxide gas is the basis for certain symptoms, it does warrant a medical consultation. Any test value greater than 10 percent warrants medical attention, even if no symptoms are evident. Carboxyhemoglobin levels ranging around 10 percent can be the cause of chest pains, leg cramps—especially at night—and shortness of breath even while resting. It should also be assumed that if one or two family members have a high concentration of carboxyhemoglobin, all members in the same environment (possibly with a faulty heater) could be so affected. Children seem to show symptoms with lower CO concentrations than do adults. If the test is positive as an apparent result of exposure at one's place of work, especially if there is reason to suspect CO poisoning, it is even more probable that all in the same environment will be affected.

Smokers who show elevated carboxyhemoglobin levels and know they are not exposed to carbon monoxide gas from any other source will find that their carboxyhemoglobin level will decrease almost immediately after stopping smoking; within a short time of being a nonsmoker (and not exposed to smokers in the immediate vicinity), their carboxyhemoglobin level will return to close to 1 percent. (Incidentally, it takes only 30 parts per million of carbon monoxide in the lungs to cause a 10 percent level of carboxyhemoglobin in the blood.)

NOTE: Sudden deliberate or accidental carbon monoxide intoxication—to the point of unconsciousness—often turns the skin bright red; the pupils are usually dilated; the breathing is more like snoring; the pulse is fast and hard, each beat seeming sharper and more hammerlike than usual. Obviously, immediate emergency medical attention is mandatory.

BREATH ODOR AND SPUTUM

The odor of one's breath (sputum related to disease is the primary source of unpleasant breath) can offer many clues to internal disease. To be sure, a mouth reflecting poor oral hygiene (see Miscellaneous Tests, **Dental Plaque Disclosure** test) can give off an unpleasant smell (see Brain and Nervous System Tests, **Smell Function** test), but proper brushing and cleaning will usually eliminate the offensive odor almost immediately. Disease-reflecting odors, on the other hand, can exist with good mouth care and usually will not disappear after brushing, albeit they may be masked momentarily by a strong mouthwash or overpowering food or drink. Certain drugs such as lithium, antifungal medicines and DMSO (dimethyl sulfoxide) can cause unpleasant breath; check with your doctor or pharmacist. Recognition of certain breath odors (not always an easy task on oneself), along with careful observation of one's sputum, can detect early warning signs of allergies; diabetes; heart, liver, lung or kidney disease; sinusitis; and even stomach lesions.

Sputum is, of course, the mucus secretion from the lower respiratory system (lungs, bronchi, trachea and larynx), sometimes called phlegm; it is the primary source of breath odor. Secretions from the nose, throat and sinuses are from the upper respiratory system and are not considered part of sputum. Sputum is usually obtained by coughing, and while it is most often cultured and examined under a microscope for bacteria, fungi or cancer cells, the amount, consistency, tenacity, color and odor of sputum can also offer clues to heretofore hidden pathology. The sputum produced right after awakening is usually revealing, but the total amount collected over a 24-hour period is best.

What Is Usual

Breath should have no distinctive odor (other than odors derived from prior intake of foods, beverages, cleansing agents, tobaccos or even chewing gum).

The production of sputum is not common, but even a healthy person sometimes coughs up small amounts. This could be a normal response to environmental irritants such as smog or inhaled chlorine fumes; in such instances, it is usually a small amount (no more than a teaspoonful a day), clear (unless slightly contaminated with soot), watery, colorless and without odor.

What You Need
A clean, dry paper cup-like container, large enough to hold all your sputum for a 24-hour period; some doctors advise two paper cups: one for sputum produced on awakening and for the first hour that follows, and the second for sputum produced the rest of the day. Do not use Kleenex-type paper tissues, for they can mask sputum characteristics.

What to Watch Out For
If you are not sure whether your breath is odoriferous, do not hesitate to have a relative or friend test you. Do not attempt to hide any breath odor with mouthwash or other artificial disguises.

Do not fail to keep a record of how much sputum you produce at various times during the day along with any possible provocative incidents that occurred (bad air quality, dust, physical activities, body position). Do not confuse expectoration (spit), saliva or nasal secretions with sputum; do not let these substances mix with sputum.

What the Test Results Can Mean
A foul breath odor, while often the result of poor mouth care, dental problems or sinusitis, can also be the first indication of a lung infection or a stomach tumor (blocking the easy passage of food), especially if it follows several days of constipation; it may even indicate cancer or leukemia. It warrants medical consultation. Acetone may be noticed on the breath before it appears in the urine and can be an important warning sign for people with diabetes; it warrants medical attention. It could, of course, also indicate that you are on a reducing diet involving intake of very few or no carbohydrates or that you have been fasting for several days. An ammonia odor could be the first sign of kidney or liver disease, and it, too, warrants medical attention.

The production of large amounts of sputum (more than one or two tablespoonfuls a day) is not normal; it alone warrants medical consultation. If sputum production is markedly increased the first thing each morning, it usually means drainage of infected or allergic lung areas by gravity: The shift from lying down to standing allows different portions of the lung to drain any overabundance of secretions. If sputum is thick, stringy and tenuous but clear, it is usually an allergic response, such as with asthma; if you are not already under medical care, it warrants a consultation. If thick but colored, it most often signals a lung infection: Green, yellow, pink or rust-colored sputum often accompanies various forms of pneumonia and industrial lung irritation; foul-smelling sputum could mean a lung abscess; red or red-streaked sputum most often means blood. All such warning signs are sufficient to warrant immediate medical attention, especially if you are taking anticoagulant drugs.

A frothy-type sputum, often pink-colored, usually comes from heart failure and the lung edema (excess fluid) that results from the heart's inadequate performance. Usually, breathing difficulties have already necessitated medical attention, but if not, bubbly, watery-pink or red-tinged sputum certainly warrants it. Should you ever notice little pieces of calcium–like particles in your sputum (somewhat like tiny shaved bits of chalk), it could be the first indication of a fungus infection of the lung or the consequence of exposure to certain minerals such as coal or silicone; it warrants a medical consultation.

SKIN SALTINESS

Cystic fibrosis is an inherited condition that, 30 years ago, rarely allowed children to live past 5 years of age. Today, if diagnosed early enough, a nearly normal life span is possible. Although it is primarily a disease of the pancreas (whose fluids help digest and metabolize foods) and other glands and tissues that excrete fluids, its most severe effect is on the mucus of the lungs, and it is now considered more of a pulmonary disease. While there are several early signs of the disease, most of these are often attributed to something else: Foul-smelling bowel movements are attributed to feeding problems, suspected food allergies and the introduction of new foods to the baby's diet; a potbelly to a good appetite and increased food consumption; stomach cramps to occasional constipation; and a chronic cough to a supposed family tendency toward allergy or catching colds easily. As a child gets older, the disease seems to concentrate on the lungs, where extremely thick, sticky mucus (sputum) plugs up the airways and causes all sorts of respiratory troubles. Wheezing and almost continuous coughing are the primary symptoms. But most of all, there is an unusual amount of sweating, and the sweat of an individual with cystic fibrosis contains much more salt than usual—so much, in fact, that it has been known to corrode metal and ruin any leather goods with which it comes in contact. While the diagnosis is usually made by precise laboratory evaluations of the sodium and chloride in the sweat, one of the earliest and simplest techniques to help detect this condition is the skin saltiness test. All that is required is to regularly kiss the cheeks or forehead of an infant—daily, and at different times of the day, for the first few years of growth. If at any time the skin "tastes" unusually salty, it warrants medical attention.

What Is Usual
Normal skin, especially in a cool room and not following any physical activity, should have no salty taste at all.

What You Need
A willingness to express affection for your child in a physical manner and a reasonably normal sense of taste (see Brain and Nervous System Tests, **Taste Function** test).

What to Watch Out For
Any unusual bowel and/or lung problems in an infant without skin saltiness that may seem minor but cannot be easily explained also warrants a medical consultation.

What the Test Results Can Mean
Performing the test can result in the early detection of cystic fibrosis, which can allow proper treatment and a reasonably normal life. It has been suggested that if every infant were tested for skin saltiness, cystic fibrosis might be totally eradicated.

HEART AND CIRCULATION TESTS

BLOOD PRESSURE

The term *blood pressure* generally refers to the pressure in the arteries as opposed to the veins. To take one's blood pressure is to measure the pressure (tension) of the blood within the artery walls. (Pressures in the capillaries and veins are quite different.) The end result is derived from a number of factors: the force of each heartbeat, the elasticity or resilience of the walls of the artery, the amount of blood flowing through the arteries at any one time, the viscosity (thickness) of the blood, the number of molecules of various substances (such as protein and sodium) in the blood, the amount of certain hormones and enzymes (such as adrenalin from the adrenal gland and renin from the kidneys) circulating in the blood, and the functioning of the autonomic or sympathetic nervous system (over which a person has no direct control) in response to changes in posture, stressful situations and other stimuli. (See Heart and Circulation Tests, **Cold Pressor and Finger Wrinkle** tests.)

Every day your heart pumps 2,000 gallons of blood through 70,000 miles of blood vessels. The blood pressure is altered during every heartbeat, reaching its highest point when the heart muscle is most contracted (forcing blood into the arteries) and its lowest point when the heart muscle relaxes after each heartbeat. The heart muscle contraction is called systole, and the medical term for the highest point of one's blood pressure is *systolic*. The momentary resting phase of the heart is called diastole, and the low point of one's blood pressure is known as *diastolic*. The difference between these two pressures is called the *pulse pressure*.

The measurement of blood pressure is really the measurement of how much pressure must be applied around an artery to close off its circulation. This is most commonly done by applying a cuff or sleeve around the upper arm and then inflating that cuff with air to put sufficient pressure on the brachial artery (the largest artery that runs down the arm) and its surrounding skin and muscles to close it off. The amount of pressure is determined from an air pressure dial, through digital display or by noting how high a column of mercury is pushed up a calibrated glass tube. The latter is considered the standard against which all other measurements are compared, and blood pressure readings are usually reported in millimeters of mercury (mm Hg), no matter what technique is used. When closure or collapse of the brachial artery occurs, the pulse can no longer be felt at the wrist or heard through a stethoscope or other electronic sound detector placed on the inside of the arm in front of the elbow. As the pressure is gradually reduced by allowing air to escape from the cuff, the point where the pulse is once again detected is recorded as the systolic blood pressure. The pulse will continue to be detected as long as sufficient pressure is applied from the outside to cause the blood's pulsations to rebound off the artery wall. When the outside pressure becomes low enough so that there is no measurable resistance against the artery wall, the pulse's sound will no longer be detected (it can still be felt at the wrist); this point is recorded as the diastolic blood pressure.

Home blood pressure testing is usually limited to measurement of an upper arm, but it can be a good idea, initially, to measure the pressure in both arms and even in the upper legs, as most doctors do. Also, when first starting out to test your blood pressure, you should measure it while standing, sitting and lying down; wait at least five minutes after assuming a new position before you take your blood pressure (see Heart and Circulation Tests, **Orthostatic Blood Pressure** test). Blood pressure tests should also be performed at various times of the day—with a note as to your activities, emotions and environment. Blood pressure can change markedly—and still be normal—when you are relaxed, after exercise or excitement, after a heavy meal, after worrying or along with any anxiety-producing situation. Blood pressure will rise if you are angry. If you outwardly express your anger, your blood pressure will return to its usual level in a short time; if you hold your anger inside you, or feel guilty after expressing it, your blood pressure will remain elevated for a much longer time.

A great many drugs can cause high blood pressure (hypertension). Some of the most common include medicines to treat asthma, birth control pills and estrogens alone, certain antidepressant medications and tranquilizers, a few of the new nonaspirin products used for arthritis and even penicillin.

At the present time it is believed that large amounts of sodium (salt) in the diet can contribute to high blood pressure (see Miscellaneous Tests, **Salt Measurements** test). But because all the facts are not scientifically proven as yet, you should not severely restrict your salt intake without first consulting your physician. Some people react with elevated blood pressure when they eat a great deal of crude licorice, while others show a rise in blood pressure after drinking liqueur made of anise; it is postulated that licorice causes sodium to increase in the blood, and the sodium holds excess water in body tissues. There have also been reports that ginseng, tobacco and antacid preparations can contribute to high blood pressure.

High blood pressure also seems to run in families; children of parents with hypertension are much more prone to develop the condition. People who are overweight have a greater incidence of high blood pressure than do those who are thin. Blacks seem much more predisposed to hypertension than do whites.

And while probably not surprising, blood pressure is usually lower while you are asleep and a bit higher than usual when you are working at your job; it is almost always lower when measured at home and higher when tested in a doctor's office.

What Is Usual

The most generalized figure used as normal for arterial blood pressure is 120/80, signifying that the systolic pressure is 120 mm Hg and the diastolic pressure is 80 mm Hg when the person is sitting down at rest and relaxed. It is not unusual, however, for a person's blood pressure to vary on occasion; it can be 120/80 at one time and be 160/100 a few hours later. This should not occur more than once or twice every few months. Although blood pressure does tend to rise with age, it should stay below 140/85; higher figures point to hypertension. It should be fairly consistent (within 5 mm Hg) in both arms and legs and after standing for five minutes after having been in a sitting position.

What You Need

A sphygmomanometer—a small, portable device that has a cuff that fits around the arm, allows pressure to be inflated in the cuff and includes some sort of instrument to show how much pressure is being applied. There are many kinds of sphygmomanometers, the primary difference being how they show the pressure values:

- Those using mercury that rises and falls inside a glass tube with mm measurements engraved along the side of the tube; they cost from $60.00 to $100.00 plus from $4.00 to $10.00 for a stethoscope to listen for the sounds
- The aneroid type, which converts mm Hg into figures on a gauge or circular dial face similar to a thermometer; these come in several varieties; some require the use of a stethoscope to listen for the sounds and, including the stethoscope, cost from $12.00 to $80.00 (much depends on the length of the guarantee); others incorporate a blinking light and/or a distinct sound ("beep"), replacing the stethoscope with a built-in microphone synchronized to the sounds that would have been heard through the stethoscope, and cost from $30.00 to $100.00
- The digital type, which displays the systolic and diastolic pressures—and sometimes the pulse rate—directly. These cost from $69.00 to $200.00.

The mercury type, while the most accurate, is also the most difficult to use at home; some come with a lifetime guarantee on the accuracy of the measuring portion (not including the rubber or cloth parts). The aneroid types that require a stethoscope are the least expensive but also the least accurate. The guarantee on the gauge's accuracy can range from three months to 10 years, and the ones that do not require a stethoscope use batteries and are much better for home testing. (In general, automatic devices that do not require a stethoscope are much easier to use.) The digital type can be battery-operated and, while the most expensive, is the best for home use; most include built-in safeguards to prevent any error in technique and are usually guaranteed for only one year, because they, too, tend to need recalibration. The cuffs may be closed around the arm by cloth ties, metal hooks or Velcro; some include easy one-hand cuff application. Some have automatic self-deflating cuffs; others require the turn of a valve screw or push of a button. Only a personal trial of the various types will show you which is easiest to use in relation to cost. The digital display type has the advantage of not requiring you to watch the measurements when testing blood pressure, something that can cause anxiety and provoke a false reading.

What to Watch Out For
The accuracy of your sphygmomanometer—no matter what type—is a vital consideration. Keep in mind that when doctors' non–mercury column sphygmomanometers were tested at random, one out of every two to three gave erroneous readings. You should check your own device against a mercury column type at least once a year, and more often if you are under treatment for hypertension.

Be sure to place the cuff properly; if it has a built-in microphone, be precise about positioning it according to the directions. Be sure your cuff is big enough; it should be at least five inches wide (cover that much of your arm) and encircle the arm without strain. If a large enough cuff is not used on an obese person, a false elevated reading can result.

Do not measure blood pressure in the arm that is used to squeeze the air pressure bulb.

If you use a stethoscope, be sure there are no extraneous noises to distract you; if you use a built-in microphone, those same extraneous noises, if loud enough, could be picked up by the microphone and give a false reading.

Do not accept a single blood pressure measurement. There should be at least three different tests, on three different days, that offer a similar result; otherwise something is wrong with your equipment or your technique.

Be sure the rubber tubing, pressure bulb for squeezing air into the cuff, air valves and other parts of your sphygmomanometer that are subject to deterioration are in good condition; pinholes in the rubber, dirty valves and a worn-out cuff can cause erroneous readings.

Do not talk while taking your own blood pressure, or while having it taken; conversation tends to raise blood pressure.

What the Test Results Can Mean

Assuming you are not already under a physician's care, any consistent reading (three different times, for three different days and under different circumstances) of a systolic pressure greater than 150 mm Hg and/or a diastolic pressure reading greater than 90 mm Hg warrants medical attention. Persistent measurements greater than 140/85 warrant medical consultation, for they can be early warning signs of high blood pressure developing and should be followed closely.

High blood pressure is more of a cause than a result of heart problems. At the same time, an elevated blood pressure can also signify kidney disease, connective tissue disease, nervous system problems, lung disease and hormonal problems. If blood pressure measurements are different in either arm or in the legs (by more than five mm Hg in one arm or leg), medical attention is warranted.

Low blood pressure measurements (hypotension), below 100 mm Hg for systolic and below 65 mm Hg for diastolic, warrant medical consultation; they could come from medicines (diuretics and other drugs such as tranquilizers), but they can also come from Parkinson-type diseases, nervous system disorders and internal bleeding.

The pulse pressure (the difference between the systolic and diastolic pressure readings) should be between 30 and 40; if greater, especially without high blood pressure, it could come from other forms of heart disease, thyroid disease or anxiety and warrants a medical consultation. If the pulse pressure is less than 30, it warrants medical attention for it could be a sign of a heart valve problem or an inability of the heart to contract and expand properly.

ORTHOSTATIC BLOOD PRESSURE

There are some people who experience a slight feeling of dizziness and may even have momentary blurred vision every time they get up from a sitting position; usually the dizziness seems greater the faster or more suddenly they arise. This is called orthostatic hypotension or idiopathic orthostatic hypotension (in medical terminology, *idiopathic* usually means of unknown origin). There are, however, a few disease conditions that can also produce the same symptoms, most of which can be easily and successfully treated if detected early enough. Measurements of the blood pressure and pulse (see Heart and Circulation Tests, **Pulse Measurements**) while you are relaxed and sitting, or even while lying down, and again after you suddenly stand for five minutes, can help discern if a medical problem exists, although it can only hint at the specific cause—usually, but not always, related to the sympathetic nervous system (see Heart and Circulation Tests, **Cold Pressor and Finger Wrinkle** tests).

What Is Usual
If you measure blood pressure just prior to standing and then again right after standing, the systolic pressure usually drops from 5 to 15 mm Hg. At the same time, the pulse rate usually increases from 10 to 20 beats. After five minutes of standing, the blood pressure usually returns to close to what it was while you were sitting, and the pulse rate returns to within 10 beats of its sitting rate.

What You Need
A blood pressure measuring device (see Heart and Circulation Tests, **Blood Pressure** test), a watch or timer (a pulse-measuring device is optional).

What to Watch Out For
If you know you experience dizziness when you rise suddenly, be sure you have someone with you to prevent you from falling. In fact, this is one of those tests that it is best to perform with another person taking and recording the measurements. Do not attempt the test if you are taking any medicine to lower your blood pressure.

What the Test Results Can Mean
Should your blood pressure fall more than 15 points after you stand, this observation warrants a medical consultation if only to establish the diagnosis of orthostatic hypotension. If the pulse rate increases by more than 25 beats a minute, accompanying the unusual fall in blood pressure, it could signify an anemia, diabetes or some other hormone disorders, internal bleeding or a very rare adrenal tumor called a pheochromocytoma. If, when the blood pressure falls, your pulse rate increases very slightly or decreases, it could signify a nerve or circulation problem, or it could also be the consequence of any one of many different drugs, especially tranquilizers, sleeping medicines, alcohol or narcotics. Any pulse alteration of more than 20 beats warrants medical consultation. When there is a variation from what is usual in both blood pressure and pulse rate, it warrants medical attention.

CAPILLARY FRAGILITY (Tourniquet; Rumpel-Leede)

If you seem to bruise easily when you bump into something, it may well be that your capillaries (the tiniest of all blood vessels and the ones that connect the arteries to the veins) are unusually fragile; that is, they break more easily than they should and release blood into the tissues. Bleeding, especially under the skin, is usually described by three terms: *petechiae*, tiny dotlike hemorrhages that resemble scarlet fever; *purpura*, red-brown or blue-brown patches, larger than petechiae but usually smaller than a 10-cent piece; and *ecchymosis*, large black-and-blue bruises.

One way to test for capillary fragility is to perform a modification of the **Blood Pressure** test. Once the systolic and diastolic blood pressure readings are determined, the pressure on the cuff around the arm is set halfway between those two readings for five minutes. The pressure is then released entirely, and two minutes later the inside of the forearm of the arm that had the pressure applied is examined for petechiae. It is usual to draw a one-inch diameter circle (the size of a quarter) on an unblemished part of the forearm prior to applying the pressure and only count the petechiae that appear within that circle. This is one of a series of tests to measure hemostasis, or how well the body responds to stop bleeding following trauma (see Blood Tests, **Bleeding and Clotting Time** tests). Since a tourniquet similar to the ones used by laboratory technicians when they draw blood from the arm is often used, the test is sometimes called a tourniquet test or, alternatively, the Rumpel-Leede test, after the two German doctors who first reported the observation.

For some unknown reason, women with red hair and women over 50 years of age may show petechiae (a positive reaction) without any disease condition.

What Is Usual
Two minutes after the blood pressure cuff has been removed, there should be no petechiae inside the circle on the forearm. However, some doctors feel that up to 5 tiny spots in a man, and up to 10 in a woman are still within normal limits.

What You Need
A blood pressure measuring device, a watch and a 25-cent piece to make the circle.

What to Watch Out For
- Do not put excess pressure on the blood pressure cuff; be precise about using the midway pressure between systolic and diastolic
- Do not use a blood pressure cuff with an automatic deflating device; it will not hold sustained pressure
- Do not count the petechiae, if they appear, until two minutes after the cuff is removed
- Do not circle an area on the forearm that contains spots, bruises or other marks that could be mistaken for petechiae.

What the Test Results Can Mean

Although the test essentially measures capillary fragility, the most common cause for 10 or more petechiae to appear is thrombocytopenia (an abnormally low number of platelets); this, as well as weakened blood vessel walls, can come from:

- An inherited condition
- A secondary result of many diseases such as cancer, kidney disease, leukemia, liver disease and infections such as flu or tuberculosis
- Use of drugs, especially aspirin, but also certain antibiotics, barbiturates, diuretics and medicines used to treat arthritis, cancer and epilepsy
- Excessive exposure to X rays or radiation
- Scurvy (a deficiency of vitamin C that can occur in alcoholics and food faddists who have poor nutritional habits; see Miscellaneous Tests, **Vitamin C Body Level**)
- Simple aging; elderly people can develop purpuric spots—especially on forearms and backs of the hands—for no explainable reason.

A positive reaction (more than 10 petechiae within the one-inch circle) warrants a medical consultation.

COLD PRESSOR AND FINGER WRINKLE

The cold pressor and finger wrinkle tests, in which the hand is placed in cold and/or warm water (along with the **Orthostatic Blood Pressure** test), help evaluate the sympathetic nervous system part of the overall autonomic nervous system. The autonomic nerves operate automatically, or without any conscious or willful control. They are comprised of two opposing systems: the sympathetic, with more of an excitatory action, and the parasympathetic, with its antagonistic action (See the Cold Face Reflex Test in Brain and Nervous System tests, **Reflex Testing**). Together the two systems help control the heart rate (pulse); blood pressure; the rate of breathing; the constriction and relaxation of the bronchial tubes; the size of the pupils; digestion in, and evacuation of, the gastrointestinal tract; urination; sweating; salivation; the tears of crying; stuffiness in the nose; some physical reactions to sexual stimulation; wrinkling of the skin; and even such prosaic activities as yawning.

These nerves act primarily without the purposeful control that is employed in deliberate movement. Emotions also indirectly influence the autonomic nervous system; fear, for example, can provoke the sympathetic nerves to quicken the pulse or dilate the pupils. If you are lying in bed and hear, or even think you hear, a strange noise—as if someone is trying to break in— usually you can immediately feel your heart beat much faster and you may even begin to perspire profusely. That is how the sympathetic nervous system works. And a great many drugs can cause autonomic system reactions: Many medicines used to treat asthma can also cause a marked increase in the heart rate and a sharp rise in blood pressure; many drugs used to treat high blood pressure can cause impotence. When the sympathetic nervous system does not reflect normal activity, it can indicate heart and/or artery disease, certain anemias, some nerve disorders or infections, a few hormone imbalances such as diabetes, and even the ill effects of alcohol and other forms of drug abuse.

What Is Usual

First you should establish your usual blood pressure and pulse rate. Then, when you place your hand in a container of ice water for no more than one minute, the impulses felt by the skin and blood vessels near the skin's surface are carried through the nerves to the autonomic system, which lies adjacent to the spinal cord. The sympathetic part of the system then sends out impulses to the heart and arteries, causing the heart to beat about 10 beats faster than usual and the arteries to constrict, which raises the systolic blood pressure some 10 to 20 points. Normally, the inner wall or lining of the artery is composed of only one thin layer of cells. When the nerve impulses provoked by the ice water travel up the arm to the sympathetic nervous system, they are then transmitted from the sympathetic nervous system to all the various body organs under its control. In particular, when they reach an artery, they cause the artery's muscle layer to contract narrowing the artery's opening that carries blood. The subsequent increased pressure on the blood flow is reflected by a rise in blood pressure. (Figure 13). If an artery's inner wall is partially obstructed due to an abnormal increase of cells—such as happens with atherosclerosis—the artery opening or blood passageway is already so small that any artery muscle layer contraction causes only a slight change in the artery opening and this is reflected by little, if any, change in the blood pressure (Figure 14). After the hand is removed from the ice water, the pulse and blood pressure should return to normal within 5 to 10 minutes.

When you place your hand in warm water for at least half an hour, a different part of the sympathetic nervous system, not directly connected to the heart, reacts and should cause the skin of the fingers to wrinkle or shrivel.

What You Need

For the cold pressor test, you need a basin of ice water, preferably at 33° F (1° C), a blood pressure measuring device (see Heart and Circulation Tests, **Blood Pressure** test) and a watch (a pulse-measuring device—see Heart and Circulation Tests, **Pulse Measurements** test—may also be employed). For the finger wrinkle test, all you need is a basin of warm water, preferably at about 100° F (39° C).

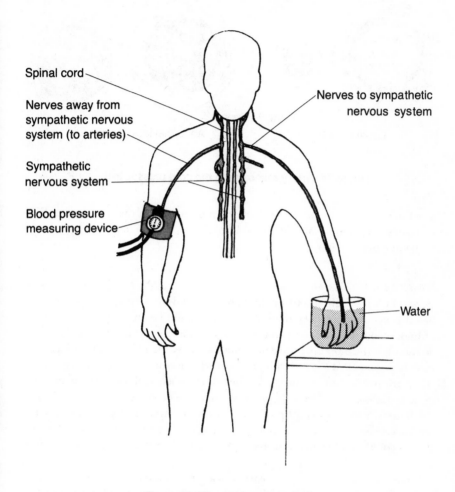

Spinal cord

Nerves away from
sympathetic nervous
system (to arteries)

Sympathetic
nervous system

Blood pressure
measuring device

Nerves to sympathetic
nervous system

Water

Figure 13. The cold pressor test.

What to Watch Out For
If you have ever had any form of chest pain, you should consult your doctor
before performing the cold pressor test; some physicians feel that this test is
quite similar to, if not better than, the exercise stress electrocardiogram test,
in that it can put an extra burden on the heart and help indicate the presence
of hidden or early heart disease. If you are over 40 years of age, you should
also discuss the test with your doctor before performing it. Do not leave your

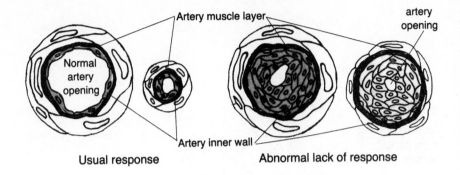

Usual response   Abnormal lack of response

Figure 14. Artery response to the cold pressor test.

hand in the ice water for more than one minute, nor in the warm water for more than 30 minutes. Measure blood pressure and pulse in the arm opposite to the one in the water.

What the Test Results Can Mean

If, within 3 to 5 minutes after the hand is removed from the ice water, the blood pressure rises more than 30 points, it could be an early warning sign of high blood pressure, and you should seek a medical consultation. If, after 30 minutes, the blood pressure does not rise more than five points or has not returned to normal (or within 5 points of what it usually is), it could indicate atherosclerosis or other diseases of the arteries such as Raynaud's phenomenon, a condition in which cold or stress can cause blood vessels—especially in the fingers, toes, ears and tip of the nose—to contract and seriously impair one's circulation. Should the cold pressor test bring on chest discomfort or pain, it could signify a heart problem. Any one of these observations warrants medical attention.

While some people with very early disease may show a usual response, any unusual response is strong evidence of something wrong within the nerve-circulation system pathways.

Should the fingers show no sign of wrinkling after being in warm water for 30 minutes, it can mean that some disease process such as Gullian-Barre syndrome—a nerve infection—might exist. Severe diabetes can also prevent wrinkling. Failure of the skin to wrinkle warrants medical consultation. Of course, patients who have had a sympathectomy—in which the sympathetic nerve chain has been surgically removed (a procedure once performed for high blood pressure or persistent leg cramps)—will never show the usual responses to either test.

PULSE MEASUREMENTS

The pulse is a manifestation of the expansion of the arteries that takes place every time the heart contracts and forces blood into the circulatory system; each heartbeat is a pulse (stroke). It is also a very sensitive reflection of the body's condition, somewhat similar to **body temperature**. Pulse measurements usually consist of rate, rhythm and character and can be obtained almost anywhere an artery lies near the skin surface; the most frequently used location is the wrist—with the palm up and two or three fingers of the examining hand resting on the artery just inside the outer wrist bone of the one being examined (Figure 15). The pulse can just as easily be counted by applying the fingers alongside the temples, along the side of the neck, on either leg just below the groin area and just above or adjacent to the protruding ankle bone on the inside of the foot (Figure 16); much depends on one's weight and excess fatty tissues, of course. Pulse rates can also be noted when measuring **blood pressure**; each sound is a pulse beat.

Pulse rhythm observations should be noted at the same time as the rate is counted; it should be regular, with no erratic interruptions or pauses (skipped beats or extra beats) after two or three rhythmic beats. As for pulse character, each beat should feel the same—none stronger or weaker than the others.

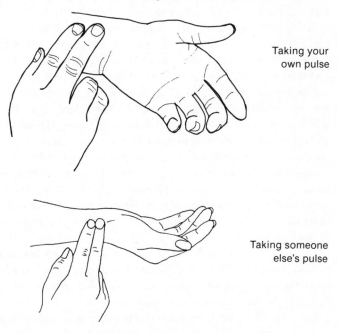

Taking your
own pulse

Taking someone
else's pulse

Figure 15. Pulse observations—wrist pulse.

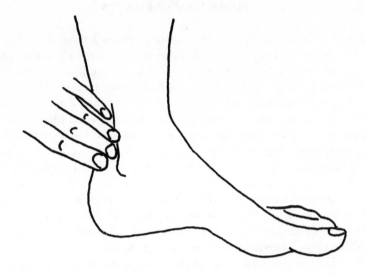

Figure 16. Pulse observations—ankle pulse.

Except when applying pulse measurements to exercise, you should sit quietly and rest for 10 minutes before testing.

When first attempting pulse measurements, it is best to count all the beats for one full minute and then observe the rhythm and character for a second full minute. With experience, the rate time can be shortened to 15 seconds and then multiplied by four.

Two-step test. One valuable pulse test is called the two-step test. You step up and down one or two steps (at least 12 inches high), at a rate of one step per second, for at least 50 and preferably 100 times (Figure 17) and note the change in your pulse rate, particularly the time it takes for your pulse rate to return to what it was before you started stepping (Figure 18). This test, which is similar to climbing several flights of stairs, makes the heart beat faster, and the heart's muscle requires much more oxygen; it is usually performed along with the **Cold Pressor and Finger Wrinkle** tests and can not only offer an early warning sign of heart or artery disease but also help indicate the state of one's physical fitness.

Note: *If you have ever had chest pains, know you have heart trouble or know you normally cannot climb a flight of stairs without difficulty, check with your doctor before trying this test; if you notice discomfort in your chest or arms while stepping up and down, stop the test and seek medical attention.*

Many people, after first obtaining clearance from their doctors to perform strenuous activity, use the pulse rate in combination with metabolic equivalents (METS) *as a means of keeping fit. One MET is considered as resting;

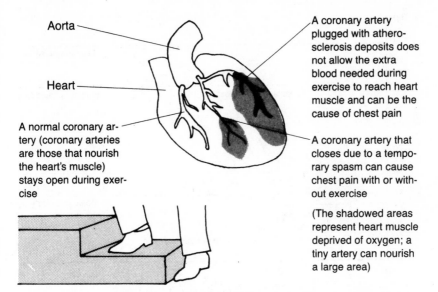

Aorta

Heart

A normal coronary artery (coronary arteries are those that nourish the heart's muscle) stays open during exercise

A coronary artery plugged with athero-sclerosis deposits does not allow the extra blood needed during exercise to reach heart muscle and can be the cause of chest pain

A coronary artery that closes due to a temporary spasm can cause chest pain with or without exercise

(The shadowed areas represent heart muscle deprived of oxygen; a tiny artery can nourish a large area)

Figure 17. The two-step exercise test.

as activities increase, the level of effort is measured in METS, depending on how much oxygen the body needs and how many calories are being burned. Your doctor can tell you your limit in METS: 3 METS—walking slowly; 4 METS—bicycling, golf or horseback riding; 5 METS—walking briskly or playing doubles tennis; 7 METS—singles tennis or skiing; 9 METS—running fast or handball; from 10 to 15 METS—very fast running (greater than marathon speed) or competitive sports. Your resting pulse rate, how much faster it becomes during exercise and how quickly it returns to normal help determine the limitations on physical activity.

Training effect. Once you are cleared for physical activity, pulse measurements can be used as a means of achieving maximum fitness through exercise. Your theoretical maximum pulse rate is computed by subtracting your age from 220. Optimal exercise is said to be reached if you expend sufficient energy to raise your pulse rate to at least 70 percent of its maximum and sustain that rate for 20 minutes, three times a week. You should not let your pulse rate go higher than 80 percent of its maximum. An example: a 50-year-old man would have a maximum pulse rate of 170 (220 − 50 = 170). Seventy

*Technically, a MET is related to the amount of oxygen consumed or used while performing various activities. It is based on the concept that the amount of exercise an individual can perform is limited by that person's breathing ability and pulse rate; it also takes the person's weight into account: 1 MET = 3.5 mL (milliliters) of oxygen use per minute for each kilogram (2.2 pounds) of body weight.

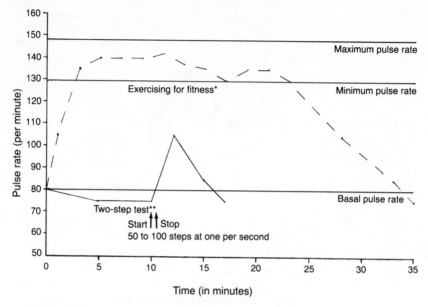

*To be performed only after medical clearance from your physician

**Not to be performed if you have chest pains, cannot climb stairs without difficulty or if heart trouble exists

Figure 18. Typical pulse patterns for a 35-year-old individual with a basal (usual) pulse rate of 80 per minute.

percent of 170 is 119; 80 percent is 136. His exercise should be sufficiently strenuous to keep his pulse above 119 (but without exceeding 136) for 20 minutes.

Many ecological and environmental conditions can affect the pulse rate. Warmer temperatures automatically increase the rate—all other conditions being the same. Smoking, caffeine, anxiety, smog and alcohol can cause an increased pulse rate. Some of these things can also cause occasional rhythm and character changes, such as skipped beats or palpitations. The use of drugs for other conditions (medicines for asthma, antidepressants, hormones and certain heart preparations) can all increase the pulse rate as a side effect of their intended actions. Other drugs such as digitalis products, sedatives and narcotics slow the pulse rate. And someone who works at physical fitness or performs regular athletic training will usually have a much slower resting pulse rate.

What Is Usual

There is no absolute standard for pulse rate; it can vary from person to person between 60 and 90 per minute and still be quite normal. It is usually higher in women. Children may have a resting pulse rate up to 120 per minute, as may some people after the age of 60. It should be regular in rhythm, although a slight increase when breathing in and a decrease when exhaling is also considered normal. After moderate exercise for one or two minutes, the pulse rate usually increases by 20 beats and then, within five minutes, returns to what it was prior to exercise. Each pulse beat should feel as if it has the same force against the fingers as those before and after it.

What You Need
Really only a watch with a second hand or digital display time in seconds is needed. However, there are many varieties of pulse monitors that count your pulse electronically and display it constantly on a digital display. Most clip around a finger or are worn like a wristwatch and do not interfere with physical activity. These cost from $49.95 to $150.00, depending on their portability and whether they also include warning devices to inform you of inadequate or excessive activity. One pulse monitor, called The Coach, even tells you how many calories you are burning up (weight loss) and how much oxygen you are consuming; it costs $200.00 and must be worn around the chest as well as on the finger. While these gadgets are not absolutely necessary, they are convenient for anyone who plans regular pulse monitoring.

What to Watch Out For
If you have any doubt about your physical condition, check with your doctor before performing any pulse-exercise tests. Do not be surprised if your pulse rate varies 10 beats up or down when measuring; that can be perfectly normal, especially if you move about at all. Check with your doctor or pharmacist to see if any medications you are using (including those not requiring a prescription) will alter your pulse. Diuretic drugs have been known to alter the rhythm of the pulse.

What the Test Results Can Mean
If your resting pulse is regularly more than 100 or less than 60 per minute, it warrants medical attention, primarily for evaluation; a rate of over 90 warrants a medical consultation. Thyroid disease can show its first signs by altering the pulse rate: Hyperthyroidism increases the rate, while hypothyroidism slows it. Internal bleeding and/or anemia also increase the pulse rate. An increased pulse rate almost always accompanies a fever (see Miscellaneous Tests, **Body Temperature** test), with the exception of typhoid fever, psittacosis (parrot or bird fever) and Legionnaires' disease. A slower-than-normal pulse rate, unrelated to fever, can be an early warning sign of out-of-control

diabetes, brain pathology (especially tumor) or kidney disease. The pulse should be felt equally on both sides of the body and in all extremities. The inability to detect a pulse at both wrists and ankles warrants medical attention, since it could indicate a circulation problem.

If you notice that your pulse seems to disappear when you take in a deep breath, it could mean a chest problem (emphysema) or a heart problem and warrants medical attention. The pulse should increase slightly on inspiration (breathing in), but when the pulse diminishes the condition is called pulsus paradoxus.

When performing the two-step test, if you notice any chest discomfort, medical attention is warranted. If, after this test, your pulse rate does not return within five minutes to what it was prior to the test, it could be an early warning sign of heart or artery disease and also warrants medical attention. If you find you cannot complete the test, albeit you have no chest discomfort and your pulse rate rises and falls as expected, it still warrants medical consultation as to the reason for your physical weakness.

Should the pulse rate not increase when exercising, or not accelerate when rising from a sitting to a standing position, this warrants medical attention; it can reflect serious heart-nerve disease.

If your heart rhythm is not regular (you notice extra-long pauses between one or two beats now and then), it warrants medical consultation. While many doctors do not feel that this syndrome (called premature ventricular beats, because the heart contracts an extra time before it is filled with blood) is necessarily due to disease, there are heart problems that can also cause the same "skipped beats," or "flip-flops." Anxiety, heavy smoking and many drugs can also cause an irregular rhythm. If the character of your pulse does not seem consistent, this warrants medical attention, for it can be the first sign of serious heart disease.

TOURNIQUET TESTS FOR VARICOSE VEINS (Trendelenburg; Perthes)

While varicose or dilated veins are usually quite obvious, especially in the legs, they can come about from several, seemingly unrelated causes, the most common being pregnancy, injury, infection and tumors within the abdomen. They usually cause symptoms such as leg aches, cramps, pains, itching, dermatitis, pigmentation, ulcers and edema (see Miscellaneous Tests, **Edema** test).

What must always be considered, no matter what the cause or the nature of the complaints, is whether the deep veins (surrounded by the leg muscles) and/or the superficial veins (just under the skin) are involved, and whether the tiny veins that connect the superficial veins to the deep veins and the valves inside the veins that control the direction of blood flow are inadequate. Without this information, treatment—especially surgery or sclerosing injections—can be a painful waste of time and money. For if the deep veins cannot properly return blood when standing or sitting, specific treatment of the superficial veins will usually fail.

The Trendelenburg test is performed by lying down, raising the leg to be tested up in the air so that all the blood in the veins is emptied out of the leg, applying a tourniquet around the upper portion of the thigh (to prevent immediate refilling of the veins from above) and then standing up. The Perthes test is performed by applying the tourniquet around the leg while standing with the veins full and then walking around with the tourniquet on for several minutes. The tourniquet, most commonly a wide piece of Velcro or rubber that can easily be wrapped or tied around the leg, can be applied at various levels of the leg to help determine whether all or only some of the veins are incompetent.

What Is Usual

Obviously, varicose veins in themselves are not normal. With the Trendelenburg test, if, after applying the tourniquet to the thigh and then standing up with the tourniquet still in place, the superficial varicose veins reappear by filling slowly from the bottom up (in about 30 seconds), this usually means that the deep and connecting veins are probably adequate and treatment has a reasonable chance of success. After 50 to 60 seconds, the tourniquet is released, and if there is no additional sudden rush of blood to fill the leg, this helps confirm the findings. If the veins seem to fill rapidly (within four to seven seconds), from top to bottom, the deep veins are probably not competent, and removal or obliteration of the superficial veins will not usually relieve symptoms.

Results of the Perthes test are considered to indicate probable effectiveness of treatment if, after walking around for four to five minutes with the tourniquet in place, the superficial veins seem smaller or less full; this usually means the connecting veins, the deep veins and their valves are adequate. If the veins seem to increase in size after walking, it usually means the deep veins are incompetent.

What You Need

A tourniquet is required. A strong, one-inch-wide piece of elastic will do, as long as it can fit around the leg. Professional rubber tubing tourniquets cost from 50 cents to $1.00. Easily applied and removed Velcro tourniquets are available and cost from $5.00 to $7.00. An "automatic" tourniquet called the Seraket, which can be applied and removed with one hand and whose pressure can easily be adjusted, costs about $10.00.

What to Watch Out For

When performing the Trendelenburg test, do not leave the tourniquet on longer than 60 seconds. With the Perthes test, remove the tourniquet as soon as the veins seem to increase in size, no matter what the time, and do not leave it on more than five minutes. Do not attempt either test if there is any leg infection or leg pain.

What the Test Results Can Mean

For home use, the tests are primarily to ascertain if surgery or sclerosing (injection treatments) will be likely to succeed; it is more of a confirmatory procedure. In many instances the use of elastic support stockings or pantyhose may be the only possible treatment to relieve symptoms. It is believed that if elastic supports are used early enough, the condition can be prevented from progressing, and subsequent therapy, if utilized, will be more successful. Varicose veins, once they appear, warrant medical attention to find the specific cause; many times, removal of the cause also eliminates the varicose veins.

EYE AND VISION TESTS

VISUAL ACUITY

Tests of visual acuity (vision) measure the ability of each eye to perceive the size and shape of an object at standard distances. They also measure the ability of both eyes, working together, to discern the distances and depths of objects and their relationship to one another (which object is nearer or farther away); this is called stereopsis, fusion or depth perception.

The most common vision test uses the Snellen chart, in which the individual is asked to read rows of distinct boldfaced letters of various sizes at a distance of 20 feet (Figure 19). For those who cannot read, there are charts that show the letter E in various positions (⊢ ∃ ⊣) or use figures such as a house, an animal, an apple, an umbrella; the positioned Es and the figures range from 3/16 inch to 3½ inches in height, with it being considered normal to see a 3/8-inch letter clearly at 20 feet. This is recorded as 20/20. The first figure indicates the distance of the chart; the second shows the line containing the smallest figures that could be read by someone with normal vision at a distance designated by the line. Thus, 20/20 indicates the ability to read the "20" line at 20 feet; 20/40 means that at 20 feet the individual could only read a line that someone with normal vision could read at 40 feet; and 20/200 means that the person being tested could only distinguish the large letter that normally could be read at 200 feet. For near vision an individual should be able to read typical newspaper print at a distance of 14 inches.

Astigmatism is an inability to see and discern letters in one plane; for example, when looking at a clock, visual acuity could be normal (20/20) for all numbers except those that would form a straight line from the 11 to the 5, which might seem blurred or darker than the rest.

Tests of visual acuity should be performed at least twice a year. An infant's vision can be checked by holding up a rubber ring to see if it is grasped; first test both eyes, then cover each one and test the uncovered eyes separately. **Pupillary Reflex** tests can also offer clues about an infant's vision. Some form of the Snellen chart can be utilized from the age of 3½ on. Observation of the pupils to see that they both seem to focus on the same point, rather than one looking in a different direction from the other, will help detect strabis-

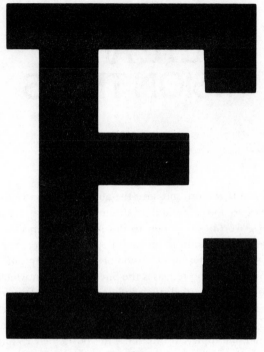

20/200

ECFDP

20/40

PODEFTEC

20/20

Figure 19. Visual acuity testing chart.

mus, which causes a loss of depth perception (see Eye and Vision Tests, **Strabismus** test). After the age of 40, it is good preventive medicine to check your vertical line perception once a month. With one eye closed, or covered, look at a telephone, flag or lamp pole with the other eye; it should look perfectly straight up-and-down.

The legal definition of blindness is 20/200 vision or worse with the use of the most efficient corrective lenses.

What Is Usual
Although 20/20 vision is considered normal, up to 20/40 vision, without the aid of glasses, is also considered within normal limits, and most states will issue a driver's license without requiring corrective lenses. You should be able to read fine print ⅟₁₆ inch high at from 12 to 14 inches (the print in this book). It is considered usual, however, to lose some near vision after one reaches 40 years of age, as the muscles in the iris lose some of their strength and cannot perform accommodation (see Eye and Vision Tests, **Pupillary Reflex** test). You should also be able to look at two objects, one in front of the other, the farther about 10 feet away and the nearer 5 to 7 feet away, and know which one is in front and approximately how far in front it lies. When looking at an astigmatism test card 20 feet away, the lines should seem uniformly dark (that is, none of the lines should seem lighter or darker).

What You Need
The Snellen charts cost from $2.00 to $4.00 and are most convenient. Printed cards to reveal astigmatism cost about $3.00 but can easily be made by drawing a one-foot-diameter circle and then drawing three parallel lines ⅟₁₆ to ⅛ inch thick from where the numbers on the face of a clock would connect (from 12 to 6, from 3 to 9, etc.) (Figure 20). You can use Figure 20 if you hold it two feet away but it is not as accurate as the full-sized card. A piece of firm cardboard with a pinhole in the center is also needed.

What to Watch Out For
Have sufficient light on the eye chart but without any glare. Keep in mind that these eye tests are only for screening purposes; some doctors feel that the Snellen chart tests are too sensitive, especially for children, and can indicate visual defects where none really exist.

What the Test Results Can Mean
The inability to read fine print when held 12 inches from the eyes or to see Snellen chart letters labeled 20/40 without the aid of lenses usually indicates a visual defect. If you look at the same letters through a pinhole and they seem clearer, this usually means that a prescription lens will improve vision. Although there is still some debate on the matter, many doctors believe that the sooner visual defects are discovered and treated, the less chance they have

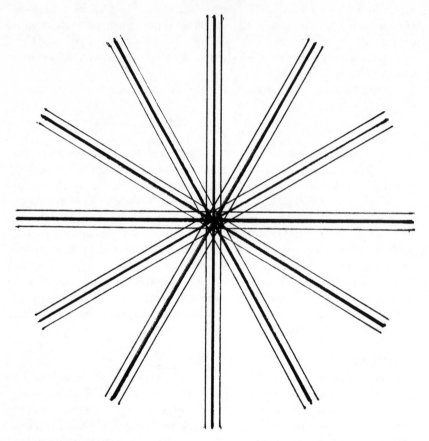

Figure 20. A sample astigmatism test chart (the lines should be 12 inches long and 1/8 inch thick).

of progressing; it has also been claimed that wearing hard contact lenses will stop the progression of myopia, or nearsightedness. Thus, any variation from normal visual acuity warrants a medical consultation. If there is obvious deviation of one eye (it may only be intermittent), crossed eyes or squinting of one eye, these are signs of strabismus, and medical attention is warranted.

If, when looking at a vertical pole, it seems bent, curved or not intact (some segments missing), it could be an early warning sign of glaucoma, cataract or retinal problems and warrants medical attention.

VISUAL FIELD

Visual acuity is the ability to see an object directly in front of you (see Eye and Vision Tests, **Visual Acuity** test). Visual field measures the eye's ability to

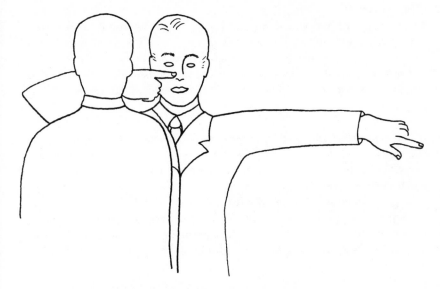

Figure 21. Visual Field Observations.

see other objects within the periphery of one's line of vision—being aware of something or someone off to the side, above or below, while staring straight ahead. While both tests help evaluate the eye and the nerves that serve it, visual acuity tells more how the lens of the eye works, while the visual field test helps assess the performance of the structures within the eye and aids in locating just where eye, eye-nerve or brain problems are located. It is quite possible to have a markedly diminished visual field and still have normal visual acuity. Home visual field testing is only rough screening, but it can be very valuable in offering early warning signs of disease.

What Is Usual
If you stare at a point about three feet away from you with one eye (the other eye covered), you should still be able to see an object that comes within the circumference of an area formed by your eyebrow, the bridge of your nose, your foot and to your side about as far back as your ear. The easiest way to check these peripheral fields is to sit opposite someone, with your noses about three feet apart, close your right eye while the person opposite closes the left one, and while staring at each other's nose (a finger pointing toward the examiner's nose helps concentrate the examinee's attention), both should see a moving fingertip or bright object at the same location in the periphery on the same side as the open eyes (Figure 21). Repeat with the opposite eyes.

What You Need
Nothing is required, other than patience and the willingness to keep staring at one point (your partner's nose) while performing the test.

What to Watch Out For

The tendency to shift your eye toward the moving fingertip or object rather than stare straight ahead. There is a small area, just off center and to the side where the fingertip will not be seen; this corresponds to the eye's "blind spot," or the place where the optic nerve goes from the back of the eye into the brain and contains no vision receptors. It is a normal phenomenon.

What the Test Results Can Mean

If you find places where the person opposite you can see the fingertip but you cannot, you should then repeat the test with someone else. If the same visual field defects remain, medical attention is warranted (and, of course, a much more precise visual field examination). Visual field defects can come from glaucoma (tunnel vision, where only objects straight ahead can be seen), brain pathology (most often a tumor), nerve involvement, infections, inherited eye diseases, hemorrhages and drug poisoning—arsenic, methyl alcohol, quinine, excessive smoking (nicotine poisoning).

COLOR BLINDNESS

About one in every 25 men (and one in every 250 women) cannot perceive the difference between red and green. This condition is almost always inherited. And there are a few people who cannot tell the difference between blue and yellow. People in many occupations require absolute color discrimination: airline pilots, truck drivers, electricians, police officers, fire fighters and military personnel. While there are professional color charts to test for color vision, it is almost as easy to screen individuals by using skeins of colored yarn, braiding together rose, red and green strands and yellow, blue and violet strands and asking the individual to separate the red or green strand from the braid. Another form of the test is to request that three different-colored strands of yarn from one braid be matched to the same color in a different braid.

What Is Usual

No matter how mixed up several colors are, an individual with normal color vision can discriminate not only between colors but between shades of the same color.

What You Need

Colored objects such as yarn skeins; colored blocks or colored paper circles will do as well, but they should have similar shapes. You should have two or three shades of red, green and pink or rose for the one test and various hues of blue, yellow and purple for the other. If color vision testing is critical,

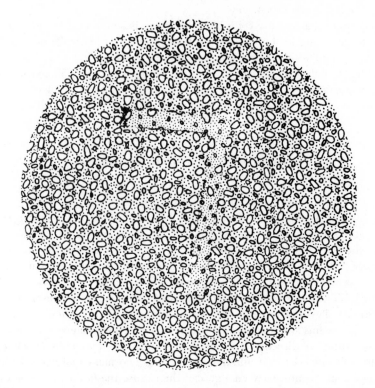

Figure 22. Color blindness observations. Although the actual color chart is made up of many different-colored dots, you should be able to distinguish a number (in this case, a 7) "buried" among the contrasting colors.

Ishihara or Hardy-Rand-Rittler color plates, in a book, are available; they cost from $5.00 to $50.00, depending on how many different plates are needed. These plates show various shades of the primary colors in various dots to make up a numeral or shape, such as a triangle or circle, and are superimposed on a background of similar dots with both contrasting and similar, but not identical, colors (Figure 22). Someone with normal vision can easily detect the number or figure within the many colors; someone with color blindness will see nothing definite.

What to Watch Out For
Some people memorize the color plates in order to avoid detection. Do not confuse color ignorance, where subtle shades of one color are difficult to name, with color blindness. Color ignorance can be corrected through education.

What the Test Results Can Mean
Being aware that you are color blind can be sufficient to enable you to learn how to get along in the world (with traffic lights red is usually on top, for example), and with practice it is sometimes possible to learn to distinguish shadings to help identify colors. If you do happen to have a blue-yellow defect, it warrants medical consultation to ascertain that the problem is not a consequence of alcoholism, along with other consequences of this disease.

STRABISMUS (Cover-Uncover; Red Dot)

Strabismus is a condition in which the two eyes do not see the identical image (see Eye and Vision Tests, **Visual Acuity** test). But unlike the usual causes of an inability to see clearly because of the shape of the eyeball (which may have been inherited) or a defect in the shape of the lens of the eye, this condition is most often due to weakness in one or more of the six muscles that control the movements of each eye. It is the most common cause of diplopia (double vision). Children usually show crossed eyes (where one or both eyes look inward) or walleyes (where one eye looks outward). The problem is that, as the condition begins and progresses, the child may not always show one eye looking in a different direction from another. A child with this condition will tend to use only one eye to see, and that eye may have normal visual acuity. Failure to detect strabismus early enough can then cause the other eye to become "lazy" and fail to develop proper vision functions; in essence, it becomes blind. Early detection of strabismus can allow treatment by eye exercises (orthoptics) and/or eyeglasses instead of surgery. Double vision can also occur in the elderly, but this is more often due to a nerve involvement.

What Is Usual
If you stare at an object 20 feet away, both eyes should be directed at the same point. When one eye is covered and then uncovered while staring, the covered eye should not shift its position. If you place a red-colored glass in front of one eye and then look at a flashlight about two feet away with both eyes, you should still see only one light.

What You Need
A flashlight and a piece of red-colored glass.

What to Watch Out For
When testing children, it is sometimes difficult to hold their attention; try and make it more of a game than a test.

What the Test Results Can Mean
If, when covering and uncovering the eye while staring at a distant point, the covered eye moves in any direction, this provides reasonable grounds for assuming that there is an eye muscle problem; medical attention is warranted. If, when looking at the flashlight with both eyes, one covered with a red glass, two distinct lights are seen—one red and one white—it is evidence of diplopia and also warrants medical attention.

PUPILLARY REFLEX

The pupil of the eye is the opening in the very center surrounded by the colored (pigmented) circle called the iris. Within the iris are muscles that can tighten or relax, thereby causing the pupil to dilate (enlarge or widen) or to constrict (contract or shrink down). The two functions originate in two different areas: Dilation comes from the sympathetic nervous system (see Heart and Circulation Tests, **Cold Pressor and Finger Wrinkle** tests), while constriction comes from the brain. Abnormal reflexes can reflect several illnesses as well as the presence of several drugs. The pupillary reflex can be tested by observation, light stimulation and by altering the distance of an object for the eyes to see.

What Is Usual
On observation, both pupils should appear to be same: round, regular in shape and equal in size (Figure 23). In a normally lighted room they should not appear unusually large or tiny. When a bright light (a flashlight beam) is directed toward the eyes or when going into bright sunlight, the pupils should contract (called miosis) and appear very small. In contrast, when the amount of light diminishes or is removed from the eye, the pupils should dilate, or widen (called mydriasis). If light is directed to only one eye, with the other eye completedly protected from the light source, that other eye should also contract (called a consensual reaction). There should be no pain or discomfort in either eye when a bright light is directed at one eye while testing consensual reaction.

When an individual looks at an object close up, within four to six inches, the pupils should contract (called accommodation). Pupillary reflex reactions should be prompt, but with aging the reaction time may seem slow and still be normal.

If you are taking certain drugs such as those used to relax the bowel (antispasmodics); antidepressant drugs; drugs used to treat Parkinsonism; drugs to treat asthma, allergy or sinus, such as adrenalin or phenylephrine; stimulants such as amphetamines or cocaine, the pupils may stay enlarged for a

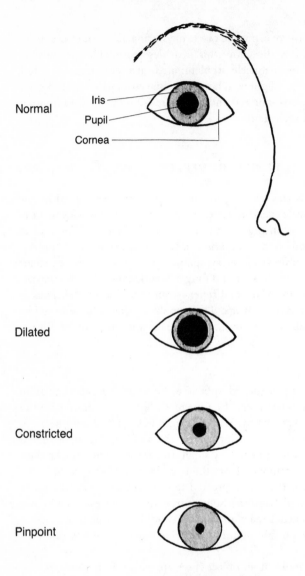

Figure 23. Pupil Size.

long period of time. If you are taking neostigmine preparations to treat myasthenia gravis, to help stimulate the bladder and sometimes to alter heart
rhythm; sedatives such as alcohol, barbiturates or chloral hydrate; or narcotics such as morphine, the pupils may stay constricted for a period of time.
Barbiturates and alcohol may also cause dilation at times.

What You Need
The test just requires a good flashlight with a bright beam (a penlight seems best).

What to Watch Out For
Primarily you should take into consideration the use of drugs (including non-prescription products) that could interfere with the pupillary reflex; if you are taking medicine, check with your doctor or pharmacist to see if it affects the pupils' reactions.

What the Test Results Can Mean
While unequal pupils (one larger than the other) may be normal in some people, it is significant enough to warrant medical attention in order to rule out any disease. It could signify brain disease, nerve disease, artery disease, glaucoma or infection—not just of the eye whose pupil is enlarged, but a generalized infection as well. Unequal pupils can also be a grave sign following an injury. An irregularly shaped pupil, where the iris edge is not perfectly round, usually comes from an old eye infection. If one or both pupils do not react (constrict) when light is shined on them or when shifting focus from a far to a near object, it could mean a generalized infection or brain pathology, or it could even hint at lead poisoning; this, too, warrants medical attention. One particular pupillary reflex condition is the Argyll-Robertson pupil, in which the pupils do not react to light but do react to accommodation; it is considered a classic sign of syphilis. Argyll-Robertson pupils warrant medical consultation. If, when light is blocked from one eye while being directed toward the uncovered eye (Figure 24), both pupils should react equally, or a medical consultation is warranted. If one eye is covered, and light directed to the other, uncovered, eye causes pain in the covered eye, it can indicate an infection of the iris of the covered eye and warrants immediate medical attention. Constantly dilated pupils can come from brain pathology (as a consequence of an injury, stroke or tumor), glaucoma, mushroom or carbon monoxide poisoning, intense fright, fear or manic-depressive behavior. It can also come from using drugs that help calm the stomach (atropine and its derivatives), drugs that help breathing (adrenalin and related derivatives including some non-prescription cold relief preparations), barbiturates and, of course, alcohol abuse and drug abuse with narcotics such as cocaine. Constantly constricted pupils can occur in people with a brain infection (abscess, encephalitis, syphilis), brain hemorrhage, nerve disorders, diabetes and especially in those using narcotics. In either case, medical attention is warranted. Fixed pinpoint pupils usually mean a severe drug overdose and requires immediate medical attention.

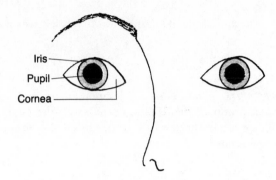

Pupillary size before shining a light in one pupil

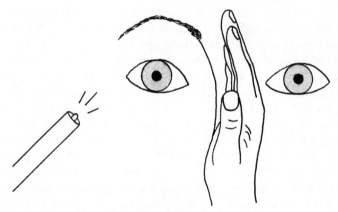

Normal pupillary light reflex reaction

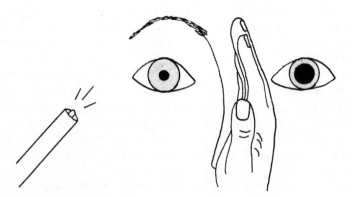

Abnormal pupillary light reflex reaction

Figure 24. Consensual pupillary reflex observation.

EAR OBSERVATIONS AND HEARING TESTS

EAR CANAL AND EARDRUM OBSERVATIONS (Otoscope)

Before any **Hearing Function** test can be performed, it is necessary to know that the ear canal is not obstructed and that the eardrum is not inflamed. Many so-called hearing problems have been miraculously cured by the simple removal of wax from the ear canal. In other instances foreign bodies such as beads, parts of toys and even insects have been found blocking hearing—especially in young children. And many ear and hearing problems arise from bacteria or especially fungus infections of the ear canal as a consequence of swimming, bathing or subsequent to scratching or picking at the ear canal. Such troubles are usually called external otitis when limited to the outer ear (from the opening to the eardrum), as opposed to otitis media, or middle ear disease, which involves the eardrum and the tiny space behind the eardrum that is connected to the back of the throat; it usually accompanies a sore throat. The third anatomical part of the ear, the inner ear, includes the nerves that transmit sound to the brain as well as the mechanisms that help keep one's balance (see Brain and Nervous System Tests, **Dizziness and Ataxia** tests).

Home testing of the ear by examination is limited to the outer ear and the outer surface of the eardrum. This is easily performed with an otoscope, a battery-operated flashlight device that projects light into the ear canal while leaving an opening for viewing (Figure 25). This instrument has replaced the once-familiar mirror with the hole in the middle that doctors used to wear on the forehead and reflect light into the ear through a speculum (a funnel–like adapter to concentrate one's vision).

What Is Usual
Once you get used to handling an otoscope, it will be relatively easy to peer inside someone else's external ear canal. As long as there is nothing obstructing the passage of the small end of the funnel tip of the otoscope, insert it carefully, always making sure nothing is in its way; if you see the slightest obstruction, you should evaluate it before continuing the examination. Without anything blocking the way, you should be able to see the pale, pink-colored

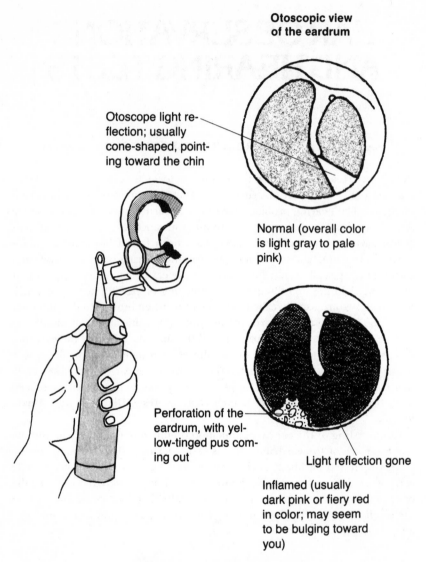

**Otoscopic view
of the eardrum**

Otoscope light reflection; usually cone-shaped, pointing toward the chin

Normal (overall color is light gray to pale pink)

Perforation of the eardrum, with yellow-tinged pus coming out

Light reflection gone

Inflamed (usually dark pink or fiery red in color; may seem to be bulging toward you)

Figure 25. Using the otoscope.

tunnel of the external canal all the way to the eardrum. The drum should also be pink, but with more of a gray tinge; most important, it should reflect your light back in the form of a triangle with the point at the center of the eardrum and the widest part toward the chin of the person being examined (Figure 25).

It is also usual to see tiny flecks of brown material along the ear canal; these most often are particles of ear wax. If they do not obstruct vision or cause discomfort when touched, they should not interfere with your view of the eardrum. If the material does not seem to be ear wax, you should not perform this examination until the foreign matter is verified professionally.

What You Need
An otoscope: They range from $17.00 for a Sears Roebuck model (which is small enough for nose examinations and also includes a lighted tongue depressor for throat examinations) to $50.00 for an otoscope only with removable speculae (funnel tips) in various sizes. Professional otoscopes cost from $70.00 up but offer no greater benefits for home use. An ear wax remover: the Murine ear wax removal system comes complete with a dropper bottle of of cleaning solution and a soft rubber syringe for rinsing; Debrox is a similar preparation without the rinsing syringe. Both cost from $4.00 to $5.00 (a generic ear wax remover that costs $1.00 a bottle is sometimes available).

What to Watch Out For
- Do not attempt or continue an ear examination if you see anything that blocks your view of the eardrum, if there is any discomfort when the speculum touches the ear canal or if there is any discharge coming out of the ear
- Do not attempt to remove any foreign body from the ear canal (other than wax, using appropriate cleaning solutions)
- Do not mistake the walls of the external ear canal for the eardrum; a normal eardrum has a distinctive light reflex
- Do not be discouraged if it takes three or four days for all the wax to be washed out; follow the instructions for the cleaning solution.

What the Test Results Can Mean
If the ear canal and the eardrum seem as they should, go ahead with hearing function tests. If the walls of the ear canal look white or red and seem to be covered with mucous, medical consultation is warranted. If the eardrum looks bulging, blue, fiery red or shows a discharge, medical attention is warranted. If, in fact, only the normal light reflex is missing or cannot be seen, that, too, warrants medical attention (Figure 25).

Incidentally, if an insect does happen to fly into an ear, a procedure that can help remove the bug is to go into a dark room or closet and shine a light into the ear; this usually attracts the insect out of the ear canal.

HEARING FUNCTION

Sound is heard and measured in two ways: by its intensity, or volume (loudness), and by its tone (depending upon how fast or slowly the sound waves vibrate). The intensity of sound is recorded in decibels (db). Loudness is influenced by distance: The same noise at 20 feet will sound 10 percent louder when it is only 5 feet away. Normally, it takes a 10 db sound to be perceived (leaves blowing in a tree just above you). Some other examples of sound intensity include:

20 db—a whispered voice near you

60 to 70 db—a spoken voice

80 to 90 db—classical music at a proper volume

110 db—thunder overhead

120 to 130 db—rock music at a typical volume

140 to 180 db—a jet engine up to 100 feet away.

Sound can cause pain at 130 db and, if heard at levels greater than 105 db continuously for 15 minutes, can cause permanent damage.

The tone of a sound is recorded in cycles per second (cps), or frequency; the lowest tones give off the smallest cps. The ear can normally hear sound with frequencies from 16 to 16,000 cps, but the typical speaking range of sound is between 500 and 1,500 cps. Frequency is also measured in Hertz (Hz) which stands for the number of pressure variations that occur per second; while similar to cps, it is said that the ear can usually hear from 20 Hz to 20,000 Hz.

Sound is perceived and conducted to the brain in two ways: air conduction (entering through the ear canal and detected by the eardrum) and bone conduction (detected by the bones around and behind the ear). It has been estimated that one out of every 10 people has some form of hearing impairment; in many cases the impairment could have been corrected or overcome had it been detected early enough in life.

Some babies, however, are born deaf as a consequence of the mothers' having contracted certain infections during pregnancy (e.g., rubella, or German measles); other infants suffer deafness as an inherited congenital defect or from injuries sustained during childbirth. While it is difficult to ascertain if an infant up to the age of 6 months can hear properly, many doctors advocate repeated home testing of a newborn's hearing starting a week after birth until evidence of hearing is observed. One such test is to sound a bell near a sleeping infant to see if it awakens at the sound. By the time an infant is 6 months old, it should have become obvious to the parents that their child does or does not respond to sounds. Another sign of deafness, albeit only partial, is failure of the child to make sounds and attempt to imitate words. It is important to be aware of any hearing defects before a child starts school; in far too many cases children have been labeled as having learning problems simply because they could not hear and comprehend words and directions.

Once a person is past 50 years of age, hearing may become impaired through aging alone, or impairment may be brought about by a hard, bony growth over the hearing bones called otosclerosis. Between infancy and aging there are many things that can reduce or eliminate normal hearing: ear infections, sinusitis and tonsillitis (although normal hearing usually returns when the infection is cured), head injuries, brain and nerve diseases, exposure to excessive noise on the job (without using adequate protective devices), and even sociocusis—a loss of hearing due to nonoccupational exposure to recreational noises (entertainment, motor boats, motorcycles, shooting, flying) or home activities (power lawn mowers, living alongside a freeway or near an airport).

A more recent cause of deafness comes as side effect of drugs. Many antibiotic medications (ganamycin, kanamycin, neomycin, streptomycin), some diuretics (Edecrin, Lasix), antimalarials, a few hormones, and even large amounts of aspirin or aspirin–like preparations are considered ototoxic (that is, they damage the ear nerves if used for prolonged periods of time). Damaged ear nerves can also cause dizziness and ataxia (see Brain and Nervous System Tests, **Dizziness and Ataxia** tests).

There are several tests that may be performed to assess hearing function; some measure sound intensity, while others evaluate tone perception or the frequency of sound heard. The ultimate test of hearing ability is performed with an audiometer—a device that can control the volume as well as the pitch (tone) of sound. While screening audiometers can be purchased for $250.00 to $300.00, it is best to apply the simple tests at home and, if problems are detected, seek out a skilled audiometer operator, who can usually define the type of deafness along with the potential benefits of treatment.

Sound Measurements. One of the simplest and most effective ways of preventing hearing disabilities is to measure and monitor the loudness of sound around you. While this can be particularly valuable in the work environment, it can be equally valuable at home if loud noises are persistently, if sporadically, present: loudspeakers emitting music; airplanes flying overhead; adjacent vehicle traffic; power tools; even some air conditioners and other mechanical appliances. Not only can loud sound damage the inner ear, it has also been reported to cause brain cell changes that, in turn, can cause behavioral changes such as confusion; some feel it is the brain reaction to damaging noises that causes ringing in the ears.

By measuring the loudness of sounds around you, and avoiding dangerous levels of sound either through insulation or wearing protective ear devices when exposure cannot be avoided, you can do a great deal to protect your hearing function. Keep in mind that repeated exposure to sound greater than 85 db is known to cause some hearing loss; and some people will lose part of their hearing at even lower decibels of sound.

What Is Usual

The voice and whisper tests are the simplest. You should be able to hear and repeat numbers spoken in a normal voice intensity from 20 feet away. Then you should be able to hear loud whispers from the same distance, and, as the whispers become softer, they should still be heard at a 2-foot distance. Whispers represent a higher pitch (tone) than the spoken voice.

Many doctors use the ticking watch test as a screening technique. Doctors know just how far away the watch must be before they no longer hear it (assuming, of course, that the doctors know they have normal hearing); they then measure the distance at which their patients are able to hear the ticking. You can perform the same three tests described, but be sure you know your hearing is normal before you test someone whose hearing is in doubt.

A tuning fork can enable you to perform a bit more refined type of test. It should have a frequency of either 512 cps or 1,024 cps. After setting the tuning fork in motion (by tapping its sides against the palm or by squeezing the tips together and releasing them suddenly), the sound should be heard by each ear at a distance of 20 feet (hold one ear closed with the palm of the hand pressed tightly over the ear against the side of the head). When the examiner compares his or her, presumably normal, hearing to that of the examinee, both should hear the sound. This is called the Schwabach test.

There are other tuning fork tests that help determine both whether air conduction or bone conduction is impaired as well as which ear is impaired. For the Rinné test (Figure 26), the vibrating tuning fork is placed next to each ear opening (air conduction); while still vibrating, the base is then placed against the mastoid bone behind the ear (bone conduction). The tone should be heard for twice as long when the tuning fork is held alongside the ear. For the Weber test (Figure 26), the base of the vibrating tuning fork is placed on the top of the head (or in the center of the forehead at the hairline), and the way each ear hears the sound is observed. It should be heard equally in both ears at the same time.

One particular tuning fork test used by doctors, but which can easily be performed at home, is the stethoscope-tuning fork test. The person to be

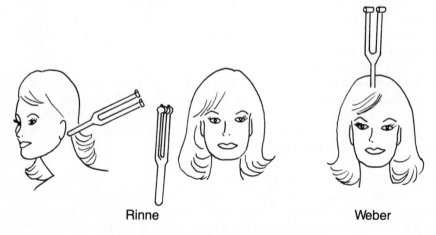

Rinne   Weber

Figure 26. Hearing tests.

tested places the earpieces of a stethoscope in the ears; a clamp can be placed over one of the two tubes that go from the stethoscope to the ears to test each ear separately. A 1,024 cps tuning fork is sounded and placed close to the stethoscope opening or diaphragm and also alongside the ear of the person doing the testing. The person wearing the stethoscope should hear the tuning fork's sound a minimum of 15 seconds longer than the person holding it next to the ear. The test is usually performed before a patient receives any drug that can cause deafness and is designed to establish a baseline time. Repeated testing during administration of the medicine and for a few months after it has been stopped can help detect deafness caused by the drug; if hearing time when the person is wearing the stethoscope is reduced by more than three seconds, additional audiometer tests are indicated.

A fifth tuning fork test is called the Teal test; it requires two tuning forks. When a person claims that the tuning fork is not heard when placed alongside the ear, the individual is blindfolded, and the base of a nonvibrating tuning fork is placed against the bone behind the ear, while another, vibrating, tuning fork is placed alongside the head about three feet away. Someone simulating deafness will claim he or she detects the sound through bone conduction; a deaf person will hear nothing.

What You Need
- An otoscope, to be sure the ear canal is not obstructed and the eardrum not inflamed prior to testing (see Ear Observations and Hearing Tests, **Ear Canal and Eardrum Observations**)
- A ticking watch or a ticking kitchen timer at $3.00 to $4.00 might be used
- A tuning fork (either 512 cps or 1,024 cps), which costs from $8.00 to $10.00
- A stethoscope (see Heart and Circulation Tests, **Blood Pressure** test)
- You might want a portable sound level meter, which detects and measures decibels; they can cost from $30.00 to $400.00 and can also offer an early warning against potentially damaging sounds. The least expensive is quite adequate for home testing.

What to Watch Out For
Be sure you check your own hearing against that of someone with known normal hearing before performing the tests. Do not perform the tests if there is wax in the ear canal or if there is any suspicion of an ear infection. Check with your doctor or with your pharmacist to see if your medicine is ototoxic. Some doctors believe mumps vaccine can also cause deafness.

What the Test Results Can Mean
Any persistent divergence from what most people can hear warrants medical consultation. Any sign of diminished hearing, especially in a child, warrants

audiometry and a professional ear examination. Any abnormal tuning fork test warrants medical attention. Two particular examples: If, when performing the Rinné test, the sound is not heard when the tuning fork is removed from the mastoid bone and held adjacent to the outer ear opening, it usually indicates an outer or middle ear problem—especially when accompanied by an abnormal Weber test. If, when performing the Weber test, the sounds seem louder in one ear, it usually means the problem is in the ear that hears the sound (as an example, perform the Weber test with your finger in one ear to block out sound). If the Rinné test is normal and the Weber test reveals hearing in only one ear, it usually indicates a problem in the inner ear that hears the sound.

Note: Part of the ear's function, in addition to hearing, is related to balance (equilibrium)—being aware of one's position in space and knowing where the parts of the body (e.g., hands, feet) are when the eyes are closed. Tests for such coordination ability (sometimes called labyrinthine tests, because the part of the inner ear that controls these perceptions is called the labyrinth) are found under Brain and Nervous System Tests, **Dizziness and Ataxia** tests.

BRAIN AND NERVOUS SYSTEM TESTS

ALCOHOLISM

The words *alcoholism* and *alcoholic* relate to compulsive alcohol dependence; they do not necessarily indicate how much alcohol is used, any particular pattern of drinking or the degree of physical damage (brain, heart and liver diseases) resulting from alcohol abuse. A skid-row type of alcoholic may take many years before alcohol abuse causes physical damage, since this species of drinker occasionally goes many days without a drink, allowing spasmodic healing. A very heavy drinker who also eats nourishing foods may forestall organ impairment for decades. In contrast, regular "social" drinking of no more than five or six cocktails a day can cause a form of alcoholism that would never be suspected by others. Medically speaking, alcoholism is said to exist when more than 70 grams of alcohol (seven one-ounce glasses of 86 proof liquor or their equivalent) are regularly consumed daily, either socially or in secrecy; *or* when blood alcohol levels above 0.12 percent (see Breath and lung Tests, **Breath Alcohol** test) do not seem to cause the usual signs of intoxication (lack of coordination, impaired functioning, drowsiness, dizziness, speech difficulties and loss of inhibitions); *or* when there are three or more YES answers to the Alcoholism Screening Test questionnaire (Figure 27) developed by the Office of Health Care Programs, Johns Hopkins University Hospital, Baltimore, Maryland (even two YES answers can, at times, indicate alcoholism); *or* if a person scores 7 or more on the Mayo Clinic Self-Administered Alcoholism Screening Test (Figure 28). A score of 7 to 9 denotes possible alcoholism; a score of 10 or greater is said to denote probable alcoholism.)

Lest you dismiss the idea that a simple questionnaire can contribute to the diagnosis of alcoholism, you should know that in a British study of several hundred people to detect alcoholics, the use of eight different laboratory tests revealed only 36 percent of those totally dependent on alcohol, while questionnaires uncovered 90 percent. Another, somewhat similar, screening program in a Milwaukee, Wisconsin hospital showed an 80 percent detection rate using questionnaires. This was more than twice as accurate as when measured against 27 different blood chemical analyses. And the Mayo Clinic's self-administered questionnaire revealed more than twice as many alcoholics as did detailed medical data without use of the questionnaire. When the Mayo

Figure 27. The Johns Hopkins University Hospital Alcoholism Screening Test

	YES	NO
1. Do you lose time from work due to drinking?	☐	☐
2. Is drinking making your home life unhappy?	☐	☐
3. Do you drink because you are shy with other people?	☐	☐
4. Is drinking affecting your reputation?	☐	☐
5. Have you ever felt remorse after drinking?	☐	☐
6. Have you gotten into financial difficulties as a result of drinking?	☐	☐
7. Do you turn to lower companions and an inferior environment when drinking?	☐	☐
8. Does your drinking make you careless of your family's welfare?	☐	☐
9. Has your ambition decreased since drinking?	☐	☐
10. Do you crave a drink at a definite time daily?	☐	☐
11. Do you want a drink the next morning?	☐	☐
12. Does drinking cause you to have difficulty in sleeping?	☐	☐
13. Has your efficiency decreased since drinking?	☐	☐
14. Is drinking jeopardizing your job or business?	☐	☐
15. Do you drink to escape from worries or trouble?	☐	☐
16. Do you drink alone?	☐	☐
17. Have you ever had a complete loss of memory as a result of drinking?	☐	☐
18. Has your physician ever treated you for drinking?	☐	☐
19. Do you drink to build up your self-confidence?	☐	☐
20. Have you ever been to a hospital or institution on account of drinking?	☐	☐

Questions © Johns Hopkins University Hospital. Used with permission

questionnaire was later compared with drunk driving arrest records and liver enzyme measurements, it proved to be 95 percent accurate. One thing all tests for alcoholism seem to have in common, whether the tests consist of blood or sweat analysis in a laboratory or a questionnaire, is that they indicate that from 5 percent to 10 percent of all people who seek medical care for reasons ostensibly unrelated to alcohol dependency are, in actuality, suffering from alcoholism. When a patient's complaints are referable to the gastrointestinal system, the chances of alcoholism being the basis for the condition rise to 40 percent.

Figure 28. The Mayo Clinic Self-Administered Alcoholism Screening Test (SAAST)*

	YES	NO
1. Do you enjoy a drink now and then? (If you never drink alcoholic beverages, and have no previous experiences with drinking, do not continue this questionnaire.)	___	___
2. Do you feel you are a normal drinker? (That is, drink no more than average.)	___	___
3. Have you ever awakened the morning after some drinking the night before and found that you could not remember a part of the evening?	___	___
4. Do close relatives ever worry or complain about your drinking?	___	___
5. Can you stop drinking without a struggle after one or two drinks?	___	___
6. Do you ever feel guilty about your drinking?	___	___
7. Do friends or relatives think you are a normal drinker?	___	___
8. Are you always able to stop drinking when you want to?	___	___
9. Have you ever attended a meeting of Alcoholics Anonymous (AA) because of your drinking?	___	___
10. Have you gotten into physical fights when drinking?	___	___
11. Has drinking ever created problems between you and your wife, husband, parent or near relative?	___	___
12. Has your wife, husband or other family member ever gone to anyone for help about your drinking?	___	___
13. Have you ever lost friendships because of your drinking?	___	___
14. Have you ever gotten into trouble at work because of drinking?	___	___
15. Have you ever lost a job because of drinking?	___	___
16. Have you ever neglected your obligations, your family, or your work for two or more days in a row because of drinking?	___	___
17. Do you ever drink in the morning?	___	___
18. Have you ever felt the need to cut down on your drinking?	___	___
19. Have there been times in your adult life when you found it necessary to completely avoid alcohol?	___	___
20. Have you ever been told you have liver trouble? Cirrhosis?	___	___
21. Have you ever had Delirium Tremens (D.T.'s)?	___	___
22. Have you ever had severe shaking, heard voices or seen things that weren't there after heavy drinking?	___	___
23. Have you ever gone to anyone for help about your drinking?	___	___
24. Have you ever been in a hospital because of drinking?	___	___
25. Have you ever been told by a doctor to stop drinking?	___	___
26. A. Have you ever been a patient in a psychiatric hospital or on a psychiatric ward of a general hospital?	___	___
B. Was drinking part of the problem that resulted in your hospitalization?	___	___
27. A. Have you ever been a patient at a psychiatric or mental health clinic or gone to any doctor, social worker, or clergyman for help with any emotional problem?	___	___
B. Was drinking part of the problem?	___	___

28. Have you ever been arrested, even for a few hours, because ___ ___
of:
A. Drunken behavior (not driving)?
B. Driving while intoxicated?
29. Have any of the following relatives ever had problems with ___ ___
alcohol?
A. Parents
B. Brothers or sisters ___ ___
C. Husband or wife ___ ___
D. Children ___ ___

Score one point for each YES answer *except* for questions 2, 5, 7 and 8; for these, a NO answer counts one point.

*A modified version of the Michigan Alcoholism Screening Test (MAST).

Early detection of alcoholism can prevent a great many subsequent serious and debilitating—even fatal—diseases, much social suffering and, when detected in women prior to pregnancy, congenital malformations in their future infants. A lack of self-awareness of alcoholism can also dangerously increase the effect of many other drugs: It can cause stomach bleeding when aspirin is used; it will interfere with the proper action of anticonvulsant drugs; it will markedly increase the sedative effect of antihistamines, tranquilizers, and other hypnotic or sleeping pills to the point where normal vision and coordination are impaired; and it can so increase the action of anesthetics as to be fatal.

What Is Usual
Not to be an alcoholic is normal. Alcoholism, however, usually is reflected in inappropriate facial flushing; dry mouth; spider angiomata over the face and chest (see Miscellaneous Tests, **Skin Observations**); a tremor of the hands; and occasional numbness in the arms, hands and feet. And as the disease progresses, there will be signs of liver and brain disease, such as the inability to remember things while still maintaining the ability to lie about not remembering; a limp wrist; a sudden increase in all sorts of injury-causing accidents, with a tendency to bleed from the slightest trauma; a hostile attitude; and finally, hallucinations (DT's) and epilepsy–like convulsions—especially if the person is deprived of alcohol for more than 24 hours. Again, all these symptoms are usual for an alcoholic, but they are not normal.

What You Need
For self-testing, you need a willingness to answer the questionnaire and face facts—admittedly not an easy option. A Spanish-language version of the Mayo Clinic Self-Administered Alcoholism Screening Test is available from Dr. Juan Ramón de la Fuente; write to the Instituto Nacional de la Nutrición, Mexico City, Mexico or telephone (905) 573–1200.

If the test is to be administered to someone else, you may need the support of your doctor, your religious leader, Alcoholics Anonymous (AA) and anyone else who might exert some influence. You will, of course, need the ultimate in patience and a willingness to uncover what brought on the problem in the first place; it might surprise you to know that it could be an inherited genetic defect or a biochemical imbalance as well as loneliness, competition, peer pressure or senility.

What to Watch Out For
What looks like alcoholism may not be; alcohol is sometimes used to cover up a totally different psychiatric problem, personality disorder or drug abuse (marijuana, heroin, amphetamines, etc.). Some forms of liver, brain and skin diseases that appear to indicate alcoholism can come from environmental toxicity, and autoimmune conditions (where the body cells make antigens and antibodies against themselves rather than against the bacteria or foreign proteins that antibodies usually fight off) can also imitate alcoholism. If the problem is alcoholism, be prepared for rebellion and an unwillingness to admit to the problem.

What the Test Results Can Mean
Unwillingness to take the test can be as obvious an indicator as a positive alcoholism score. Either warrants a medical consultation. If you seek medical help, be sure to inform your doctor as to the reasons; far too many doctors are reluctant to recognize alcoholism as a disease and tend to discount it. Do not argue with such a doctor; find another. Alcoholism can be quickly and successfully treated, and the result can mean great savings in anxiety, health and money; all can then be applied to a better life.

DIZZINESS AND ATAXIA

Dizziness seems to be an increasingly common complaint, especially among older people. The word *dizziness* can have many different meanings; medically, however, it stands for instability or unsteadiness, along with lightheadedness and a fear of an impending fall. The word is also used frequently for *vertigo*, which means either you feel the room going round and round or something inside your head seems to be going round and round. Some people use the word to describe a lack of the sense of balance, when, in fact, the problem is more a loss of coordination—usually referred to as positional imbalance. Ataxia, on the other hand, is a loss of muscle coordination or unexpected, irregular muscle actions; it is often considered as dizziness because of the difficulty in walking and position sense.

There are many totally different illnesses that can cause dizziness or ataxia, and these conditions may come on so gradually that they are overlooked until they become extremely difficult to treat. But if dizziness occurs several times, it is sometimes possible, by applying a few basic tests, to help detect the cause of the dizziness while the condition is still in its early stages.

Keep in mind that a great many medicines can, indirectly, be the cause of dizziness; they include: certain antibiotics (see Ear Observations and Hearing Tests, **Hearing Function** tests), several diuretic drugs, tranquilizers and anti-depressants, antihistamines, drugs used to treat high blood pressure and epilepsy, birth control pills, large doses of aspirin and even excessive amounts of alcohol, caffeine or nicotine. And also, new glasses, allergies and anxiety can all bring on "dizzy spells." In most instances, withdrawal of the provocative factor results in a cure. The **Orthostatic Blood Pressure** test may also offer a clue to the problem.

While it is not likely that you can make a specific diagnosis for the cause of repeated dizziness, vertigo, ataxia or positional imbalance, it is sometimes possible to help discern the problem by applying six basic dizziness and ataxia tests:

- The Romberg test—the individual stands up with feet close together, arms at sides, and then closes both eyes; be sure someone is ready to catch the person should he or she start to fall
- The past-pointing test—have the individual sit in front of you with eyes closed, holding out both hands with the index fingers pointing at you; placing your fingertips underneath his or hers, tell the person to lift up both arms over his or her head and then return the index fingers to where they were (on your fingertips, which you have kept in place)
- The finger-to-nose test—have the individual stand up and, with eyes closed, extend one arm all the way out to the side, hold it out straight and then quickly bring back the index finger to the top of his or her nose, keeping the elbow perpendicular to the body; test both arms
- The finger coordination test—have the individual touch each fingertip with his or her thumb in rapid succession, back and forth; test both hands
- The heel-to-knee test—have the individual lie down on his or her back and place the heel of one foot on the knee of the opposite leg, first with the eyes open and then with them closed; test both feet
- The toe-pointing test—have the individual lie down on his or her back and point to various objects with his or her big toe; test both feet.

The various tests can help locate the area where the problem exists: the inner ear (see Ear Observations and Hearing Tests, **Hearing Function** tests), the cerebellum (that part of the brain which helps control balance and coordination), or the spinal cord and nerves below the brain level (see Brain and Nervous System Tests, **Reflex Testing** and **Sensory Testing**).

What Is Usual
An individual should not sway or fall when standing up with the eyes closed. All the other tests for coordination and position awareness should be performed without difficulty.

What You Need
Nothing in the way of equipment; but patience and encouragement help.

What to Watch Out For
When performing the Romberg test be sure you are physically able to catch the individual should he or she start to fall. If there is a problem, be sure to ascertain that it is not drug-induced.

What the Test Results Can Mean
A positive Romberg test (falling) and past-pointing test (inability to bring the fingertips back to where they were) usually indicate an inner ear problem (see Rinné and Weber tests under Ear Observations and Hearing Tests, **Hearing Function** tests); less often it points to a loss of positional sense, with the trouble being in the spinal cord. If the foot misses its mark with the heel-to-knee test and keeps slipping down the front of the leg instead of staying on the knee, and there is an inability to perform most of the other tests, this usually signals a cerebellum disorder but can also hint at spinal cord disease. When these tests are accompanied by a staggering or lurching type of walk, they could come from an old spinal cord infection such as syphilis. In general, however, almost all of the tests are positive (there is an inability to perform them easily and properly) with: thyroid disease and other hormone disorders, anemia, some vitamin deficiencies (especially niacin or B_3), spinal cord involvement (multiple sclerosis), various forms of heart and artery disease, the late consequences of injuries, migraine and the reflection of a neurosis. Thus, it is easy to see why any abnormal test result warrants medical consultation. If, of course, the dizziness or ataxia is recurrent and close to disabling, it warrants medical attention. Sometimes, that visit to the doctor results in an immediate cure, such as when the problem is nothing more than a foreign body in the ear (see Ear Observations and Hearing Tests, **Ear Canal and Eardrum Observations**), an allergy, a form of motion sickness, or the consequence of hyperventilation or some other anxiety-type reaction.

MENTAL ABILITY AND PERSONALITY TESTING

Mental ability tests encompass a wide variety of evaluations. Although many are interrelated, different forms of these tests are intended to reveal different abilities as well as disabilities. In general, they are categorized as:

- Intelligence tests (IQ)—to estimate a person's ability to make use of learning, reasoning, social experience and memory for problem solving; these tests also contribute to understanding learning disabilities and personality problems
- Achievement tests—to evaluate the success or failure of past formal educational experiences; they are designed not simply to compare a child's academic qualifications to those of his or her peers but to uncover learning disabilities early enough for correction
- Aptitude tests—to ferret out latent talents, usually in some specific field such as art, mathematics, mechanics, music, science or stenography
- Personality tests—to evaluate an individual's social actions and adjustment to life; most often administered when a person's attitudes and behavior appear to deviate from what is considered usual.

In the past such appraisals were categorized as "psychological" tests, primarily because they were an outgrowth of clinical psychological studies. Now, however, they have changed to reflect educational and social studies equally as much as psychiatric theories. Tests that employ projective techniques (the examiner's personal decipherment) have not changed over the years and cannot be standardized by objective measurements. In the interpretation of many of these tests, responses to some questions must be filtered through the background, training and prejudices of the examiner; the consequences of such bias, whether conscious or not, allow two different examiners to observe identical responses and yet arrive at totally dissimilar conclusions.

It must be kept in mind that the results of any mental ability or personality test reflect only a sample of an individual's performance in response to a question or direction, whether written or spoken, and must never be considered conclusive. Such tests can be compared to X-ray studies. When viewing an X–ray, all that can be seen are expected shadows, possibly unexpected shadows, or a lack of shadows where they should be; the shadings and shadows do not tell a doctor the diagnosis. Rather, after many years of training and experience, the doctor interprets those shadows into logical possibilities, which still must be confirmed by concrete evidence before they have any real meaning. According to one study, two or more radiologists looking at X rays of known cancer disagreed on what the shadows meant almost 50 percent of the time. A mental ability or personality test is but one possible clue to an individual's character, individuality, qualifications, peculiarities and other identity traits.

Regardless of just how inconclusive mental ability and personality tests can be, they are an integral part of almost everyone's life. Sooner or later, you or your child will be taking one or more of these tests. Depending upon how they are applied, they can be good or bad. One thing is known: The more familiar people become with such tests, the easier they find them, for they are more aware of what is expected and are less apprehensive. Therefore, each time a test of this sort is taken, there is an increased possibility of its reflecting true intellectual and academic achievements.

Intelligence Quotient (IQ)
Although there is no universal agreement on the definition of intelligence, the present consensus seems to be that it is the ability to make use of learning, reasoning and memory in problem solving. Most intelligence tests measure an individual's ability to learn in comparison with the ability of the general population. The intelligence quotient (IQ) is expressed by dividing the mental age (as determined by the tests) by the chronological age (the individual's actual age in years and months) and multiplying the result by 100. For example, a 10-year-old with test results showing an average mental ability for that age would have an IQ of 10/10 × 100 = 100. A 20-year-old with a mental ability score equal to that of a 30-year-old would have an IQ of 30/20 × 100 = 150. Many doctors feel that this formula is not applicable after the age of 25, since some mental processes seem to diminish after the twenties are reached.

There are numerous forms of intelligence tests; some rely mostly on the individual's verbal ability (Stanford-Binet), while others also take into account physical performance (Wechsler). Performance tests are best for young children, the handicapped and people who have a limited knowledge of the language in which the test is written. Some feel that performance tests are better predictors of social adjustment, while verbal tests are better predictors of educational achievement.

Group tests such as those used by the military and schools are not considered to be as accurate as individual tests, and some states have outlawed group IQ testing. Few group tests take into account the background and environment of the individual, which can seriously distort scoring. For example, a child raised on a farm might identify a picture of a pail as a milk pail, while a child raised in the city might interpret the same picture as a champagne bucket. If the tester does not take into account the child's experiences, the child could be unfairly penalized in the final scoring.

IQ test questions are similar to the following:

* Repeat backwards: 9 – 2 – 4 – 6 – 8 (young children are given three digits; adults, up to nine digits)
* Make up a short story about a picture that is shown
* Describe how certain words are related (for example: orange, banana; or auto, train)
* Find the missing part in a picture
* Rearrange the order of several pictures to make them show a story in sequence.

Intelligence tests are no longer used as the sole determination of mental retardation as they once were. Still, they can be helpful in evaluating learning, memory and reasoning powers and in diagnosing learning disorders.

Cognitive capacity screening is a variation of IQ testing; it is used more to help distinguish dementia due to organic disease from functional delirium or an unwillingness to behave properly. Dementia is a physical disease, primarily in older people, that usually results from degeneration of brain substance subsequent to little strokes (tiny blood clots in the brain's circulation that often go unnoticed) or from atherosclerosis of brain arteries, which can accompany diabetes, high blood pressure or heart rhythm disorders; recent research seems to attribute the condition to a slow-growing virus. A lessening of intellectual functioning, especially in the elderly, can also come from drugs, liver and kidney disease, and nutritional deficiencies. The cognitive capacity test consists of asking several questions that require a certain degree of mental ability:

- Listen to these numbers—8 – 1 – 4 – 3; now count from 1 to 10 out loud and then repeat the four numbers you first heard
- Take 7 away from 100, and what do you have?
- Keep taking 7 away from each answer, and what do you have?
- What is the day of the week, the date, the month and the year?
- Who was president of the United States during World War I? World War II? Today?
- Where were you born? When? What did you have to eat for your last meal?
- Suppose you smelled smoke in your room; what would you do?
- What does the expression "Never one door closes but another opens" mean?

The failure to answer two or more of these questions correctly warrants a medical consultation regarding the possibility of brain disease or an overdose of medicine.

The *Mini-Object* test is a more refined way of screening for dementia, especially senile dementia (one form of which is sometimes called Alzheimer's disease). All that is required are 15 of the 50 or so 3½ inch long plastic miniature tools and other objects that come boxed in the game called Jack Straws (the Parker Brothers game is available in toy shops for about $6.00). Each different object (*e.g.*: shovel, saw, wrench, rake, ladder, etc.) is shown to the individual. For each object correctly identified, one point is scored. After identification of the object, or even after lack of proper identification, the individual is asked to show how the object works or how it is used. Again, one point is scored for each correct response. A perfect score would be 30 points. Individuals who have problems with abstract thinking, difficulties in sensory perceptions (see **Brain and Nervous System** tests, Sensory Testing) or beginning incoordination impairment will usually score under 15 points; any score under 24, however, warrants a medical consultation.

The *number connection test* is another form of intelligence testing used to screen individuals whose thought process appears confused. Although the test is used primarily to see if a brain problem is the consequence of liver disease (see Urine Tests, **Bilirubin** test), it can also help differentiate a physically caused learning problem from anxiety-provoked learning inabilities. A sequence of numbers, inside small circles, are place at random on a sheet of paper; they may run from 1 to 10 or even 20. The individual is asked to connect these numbers with a pencil line in correct sequence. It resembles the children's game in which a picture was formed when dots next to consecutive numbers were properly connected. Failure to connect the numbers in sequence or taking an excessive amount of time to connect them warrants medical attention.

Attempting to draw definitive conclusions about intelligence based on only one test should be considered with caution, and some courts have ruled that a person suffering embarrassment or unfairness as a result of an IQ rating can be compensated by a monetary award.

Achievement Tests

While intelligence tests are supposed to measure one's *ability* to learn, achievement tests are constructed to measure how well past educational experiences were understood and remembered. For example, reading readiness tests, usually given to children in kindergarten or just prior to entering the first grade, will reveal whether the child knows capital from lowercase letters, can recognize printed words with similar sounds and can remember words a short while after they have been taught. As a child grows older, there are specific achievement tests covering various academic subjects, such as reading comprehension, mathematics understanding and application, spelling ability and how much was learned in relation to grade standing in science, social studies and vocabulary. Most of these tests derive their questions and answers from the typical curriculum taught throughout the United States at each grade level and are based primarily on what a child should have learned for his or her age and grade. Many schools require children to take achievement tests every few years.

Until recently a child's ability to learn, especially as observed in the school environment, was considered a nonmedical condition. It is now known that a child's inability to understand and remember as well as his or her peers can result from inherited developmental disabilities causing mental retardation (see Urine Tests, **Phenylketonuria** test), eye and ear difficulties (see Ear Observations and Hearing Tests, **Hearing Function** and Eye and Vision Tests, **Visual Acuity** test), muscle incoordination (see Brain and Nervous System Tests, **Dizziness and Ataxia** tests and **Reflex Testing**), hormone disorders and even allergies (see Miscellaneous Tests, **Allergy Patch Testing and Elimination Diet**), especially those that cause hyperactivity. And there are many medicines children take for seemingly unrelated conditions that, in turn, cause impaired learning as a side effect. Dyslexia, or difficulty in understanding the written word because of a brain problem in which the child sees printed letters reversed (*dog* is read as *god*), is probably the most common learning disability. At the same time, a child can have a condition that distorts the meaning of words in a sentence, preventing comprehension, and still can excel in mathematical ability. Achievement tests, especially reading readiness tests, can be the very first indication of a learning disability in a child whose close preschool parent relationship obscured some slight mental or physical defect.

The standard achievement tests used by schools are primarily the Metropolitan and Stanford; these usually comprise several different subjects and measure learning for each year from kindergarten to the 12th grade. There are many other commercial tests to measure a child's skills in reading ability and specific subjects, and there are related tests that evaluate an adult's past academic achievements; the latter are used mostly by personnel departments prior to employing workers who did not complete formal education.

The *Bender-Gestalt test* is one specific test that measures the ability of the eye to see, the brain to understand, and the muscles and nerves to be able to coordinate and carry out the brain's directions. Here the child is shown geometric designs, from simple squares to complex patterns, and is then asked to copy them. Some examiners leave the drawing in front of the child; others ask the child to reproduce the figures from memory. How well the drawings are reproduced, taking into consideration the time it takes, can help detect a learning disability.

A simple home screening test along the same line is to show a child aged 5 or older the symbols on the aces in a pack of playing cards and ask him or her to copy them on another piece of paper. By comparing the child's copies to the originals and, if possible, to the artistic efforts of another child of similar age, it is sometimes possible to detect a learning disorder at its earliest stages and start corrective measures.

Aptitude Tests

Intelligence tests are usually general in nature; that is, they measure a combination of all one's abilities working together. Aptitude tests, on the other hand, are essentially intelligence tests that evaluate the integral fragments that comprise overall intellectual abilities. One child may have an uncanny ability to discern musical components; another, while unable to recognize a high tone from a low one, can glance at a picture of a complicated piece of machinery and immediately delineate its workings as well as notice any possible flaw concealed in the illustration. Thus, an individual could have a low IQ score and yet be a musical virtuoso or possess exceptional mechanical reasoning, both of which could be overlooked by routine IQ testing. There are individuals who fail the IQ test, figuratively speaking, and yet have exceptional powers of abstract reasoning; their creativity would go unnoticed unless deliberately sought out.

Related aptitude tests are available that attempt first to assess one's capacity to grasp unusual, ostensibly difficult training and then to foretell success in one of the professions, such as medicine, nursing, law and accounting. Most of these tests try to measure the ability to interpret offered facts, memorize them and then follow a logical sequence to a conclusion not actually stipulated in the facts. Tests of vocational interests and career planning tests also fall into this category.

Personality Tests

Unlike intelligence, achievement or aptitude tests, which attempt to measure something of a more positive nature, personality tests (now more commonly called personality inventories) are supposed to reveal negative behavioral traits and the reasons behind them. Although it has been claimed that personality inventories can differentiate between neurosis and psychosis; can specify a psychosis; can detect hypochondriasis; and can even discern sociopathic disturbances, such as sexual identity conflicts and other forms of dyssocial reactions, the usefulness of these tests has never been scientifically documented in controlled studies. Almost all personality evaluations depend not only on the examiner's interpretation but also on the honesty of the responses of the individual taking the test. For example, a test may ask if the individual wishes he or she could be as happy as others seem to be. The score for that question depends not only on what the test creators felt a "normal" response should be but also on what the person taking the test felt would be the best answer for himself or herself. It may be nothing more than a yes or no reply, or there may be a graded choice of responses, but the variables of pleasing one's self and the examiner, along with indeterminate prejudices, make an objective evaluation of personality virtually impossible.

Still, personality inventories abound, and many people are forced to come face-to-face with them for employment opportunities, educational situations, medical or psychiatric diagnosis and prognosis, or as a means of avoiding the consequences of the law. Someday you may be induced to take a Minnesota Multiphasic Personality Inventory (MMPI), where you will be given a box of 550 statements, each printed on a separate card, and asked to file them in piles as to whether you agree with the statement, disagree or "cannot say." An approximate example: "Sometimes I think my friends are talking about me behind my back." Your answers will allow an examiner to categorize you as being: normal, hypochondriacal, hysterical, paranoid, schizophrenic, homosexual, psychopathic or simply weak in the mind.

Other personality inventories range from describing what you see in smudges of inkblots to placing characters on a miniature stage (designating that stage as a house, a room in the house or simply as a theater). The names of some other personality inventories include: the Rorschach Technique (10 inkblots), the Holtzman Inkblot Technique (using 90 inkblots), the Make-A-Picture Story (using the stage setting to construct a scene), the Draw-A-Person test (where you are asked to draw one person and then a person of the opposite sex, emphasizing the "best" and "worst" parts of the body), the Thematic Apperception Test (you look at pictures and make up stories about what you think the people in the pictures are thinking; there are children's versions using animals in place of people) and the Rotter Incomplete Sentence Blank test (where you are told the first word or two of 40 sentences and asked to complete each one). These are only a few examples; all these tests are alleged to reveal your attitudes, desires, fears and wishes, thus unmasking your personality.

Some variations of personality tests include the Jenkins Activity Survey (whether you are a Type A or Type B personality; whether you are impatient, overly competitive, and time is very important to you) designed to find out if you are unusually prone to a heart attack.

The threat of privacy invasion is only one problem of personality testing; many people find such tests threatening to their self image as well. Before you voluntarily take any type of personality test, be sure you understand the reason you are being given the test and that the results will be kept confidential.

What Is Usual

I. Q. scores have been standardized by compiling the result of the testing of people of all ages the world over. In general, an I.Q. score of from 90 to 110 is considered average. Below 83, is suggestive of a slight degree of mental retardation; below 70 is suggestive of mild retardation; a score in either range warrants a medical consultation. Between 83 and 90 is considered borderline and warrants repeat testing. A score greater than 140 is considered "genius" level, and when a score is over 130, a person becomes eligible to join Mensa, the international high-IQ society, with 41,000 American members. A Wechsler score seven points lower than a Stanford-Binet score is considered equivalent.

Achievement tests are generally scored as to grade level; a child in the sixth grade should reflect knowledge equal to that attained by most children who have completed the fifth grade. Some schools require children to show they have acquired knowledge eqivalent to the seventh grade before they are allowed to graduate from high school. The Bender-Gestalt test is usually not given until a child reaches the age of 5. By the age of 7 he or she should be able to copy at least two designs, and by age 10, all of them.

There are no normal or abnormal results for aptitude testing; the individual either shows some particular talent or ability or does not.

Since virtually all personality tests require projection or interpretation, normal is in the mind of the beholder—in this case, the person giving the test. Among psychometrists (those who specialize in testing), individuals who end up with "good" scores (showing few or no abnormalities) are all too often considered overly eager to please the examiner.

What You Need

Just about every kind of test is available in books from the library or bookstore. Ask your librarian or bookseller to show you the current edition of *Medical Books and Serials in Print*; in the "Subject Index" section of that book, check for appropriate titles under the following headings: Ability—Testing, Intelligence Tests, Learning Ability, Learning Disabilities, Personality Assessment, Personality Tests, Psychological Tests and Self-Evaluation. In most instances copies of actual tests along with expected answers, scoring and interpretation are given; otherwise, reasonable facsimiles of the real tests are offered. A few titles and sources include:

- *Know Your Own I.Q.* and *Check Your Own I.Q.*, by H. J. Eysenck (these are also paperback books published by Penguin at $2.50 each)
- "The Standard I.Q. Test," obtainable by mail from Mensa Headquarters, 1701 West Third Street, Brooklyn, New York 11223, for $8.00 (it may be available locally; check your phone book for Mensa)
- Test workbooks similar to reading readiness and achievement tests are usually found in school supply stores
- "The Guided Career Exploration" test material, which reveals aptitudes in relation to career exploration, costs $160.00 for everything you need to test 25 children, including cassette recordings; single test workbooks cost $2.75, and an explanatory manual is $16.00 from The Psychological Corporation, 757 Third Avenue, New York, New York 10017
- Sample aptitude tests for almost every job and profession have been published by Arco Publishing Company, which also puts out many different achievement tests
- *Check Yourself Out* by Craig Norback—a personality test published by Times Books for $8.95
- *Adult Assessment: A Source Book of Tests and Measures of Human Behavior*, by Richard S. Andrulis—a paperback published by C.C. Thomas for $16.00
- *How to Beat Personality Tests*, by Charles Alex, published by Arco Publishing Company as a paperback for $1.45; it may be out of print but can still be obtained in libraries or through book-finding services and is well worth the effort to locate.

While a great many tests are available directly to individuals to perform and interpret at home, some must be acquired through schools, employment personnel offices, psychologists or physicians. Many are still completed at home, but a few must be interpreted by the professional tester. The largest single source of testing material is The Psychological Corporation (noted above). Other test sources can be found in the telephone company's Yellow Pages under the headings of Aptitude and Employment Testing and Psychologists.

What to Watch Out For
Your own personal bias can be a problem, as can the temptation to cheat by not following instructions to the letter or by not answering the questions honestly. Do not accept the test results at face value without considering your background, education and environment. Be sure any unusual test results are not caused by drugs, as many nonprescription products such as antihistamines and other cold preparations can dull the senses; other medicines can help bring on hypoglycemia (see Blood Tests, **Glucose** test), and even large doses of aspirin and some weight-reducing aids can cause temporary mental incapacity. Anticholinergic drugs, many of which are used to treat allergies, gastrointestinal problems and Parkinson's disease can cause memory defects.

What the Test Results Can Mean
Although tests of mental ability and personality are not considered hard evidence of a medical condition, they can suggest the need for further diagnostic investigations, especially in children with apparent learning problems. Test results that vary significantly from what is expected warrant a medical consultation. When appropriate tests were performed on patients thought to have incurable senile dementia, more than 25 percent of them showed they really had easily treatable behavioral problems. More than anything else, familiarity with such tests can prevent subsequent erroneous test result interpretations and avoid erroneous or unnecessary therapies.

BECK DEPRESSION INVENTORY

If you feel depressed at times, you are not alone. Research has shown that more than 10 percent of all patients who seek medical help through their family doctor or an internist have some form of depression. If the patient is elderly, at least one out of every three suffer from this affective disorder. Women suffer depression five times as often as men. Unfortunately, the same study that uncovered the extent of the problem, also revealed that doctors missed diagnosing depression in three out of every four of their depressed patients. In addition to this problem is the fact that even psychiatrists do not agree on precisely what depression is, how many different kinds of depression there are and just how depression, once diagnosed, should be treated.

In general, depression can take two forms, primary and secondary. Primary or endogenous depression is found most often in people over 40 and is usually accompanied by a family history of depression. The external symptoms of primary depression are:

• Insomnia
• Loss of appetite followed by weight loss
• Loss of interest in sex
• Loss of friends
• Loss of energy
• Increased brooding about death
• Guilt
• Hopelessness
• Vague aches and pains
• Increased irritability.

Most of all there is an obvious loss and avoidance of normal pleasures.

Secondary or reactive depression seems to occur in younger people with no family history of depression and rarely displays the usual symptoms of primary depression, other than sleep disorders. Secondary depression is most likely the consequence of a real or perceived insurmountable obstacle in a person's life. It is usually of sudden onset and is most often accompanied by self pity. It is often successfully treated with nothing more than empathy. In contrast, primary depression seems to be a continuing pattern in the sufferer's life.

Depression can also be manifested in many seemingly unrelated ways. The most common disguise is chronic pain in the back or the head. Or it can masquerade as stomach problems such as indigestion, ulcer-like pains, constipation, or diarrhea. It can also seem to appear out of nowhere immediately or shortly after pregnancy in spite of the joy of a new baby. When unexplainable symptoms persist and cannot be diagnosed, it is a good idea to think of an underlying depression. Observation of other family members of a seemingly depressed person can sometimes help to confirm a diagnosis of depression, for those directly associated with a depressed person usually show signs of depression themselves.

A diagnosis of depression can often be made erroneously in the presence of dementia (see Intelligence Quotient, *Cognitive Capacity Screening, Mini–Object Test*), hormone problems (especially hypothyroidism), certain forms of heart disease, with many forms of cancer and with kidney disease. Many drugs can cause a depressive reaction such as reserpine drugs used to treat high blood pressure, steroid medications, sedatives, tranquilizers, heroin, morphine, marijuana, excessive amounts of alcohol and oral contraceptives. Pills to curb one's appetite can cause depression after they are stopped as can withdrawal from cocaine use. When in real doubt, your doctor can perform the adrenal suppression test (sometimes called the cortisol suppression test) where a tablet of a cortisol-like drug is given at bedtime to see if it suppresses the body's own cortisol excretion (which it normally should). Thyroid function testing should be routine when depression is suspected, as should urine catecholamine measurements prior to any form of therapy.

It does not seem to matter whether depression is a manifestation of one's mood, a reflection of evident grief, or whether it is an overt symptom of a serious underlying mental illness. Its early diagnosis is necessary to prevent suicide attempts. There are several questionnaires that, when honestly answered, can not only point to the need for immediate medical attention but can help direct attention to some latent condition which, when treated, will eliminate the depression as well as the disease. One such test is the Beck Depression Inventory:

Figure 29. Beck Depression Inventory.

On this questionnaire are groups of statements. Please read each group of statements carefully. Then pick out the one statement in each group which best describes the way you have been feeling the PAST WEEK, INCLUDING TO-DAY! Circle the number beside the statement you picked. If several statements in the group seem to apply equally well, circle each one. **Be sure to read all the statements in each group before making your choice.**

1   0 I do not feel sad.
     1 I feel sad.
     2 I am sad all the time and I can't snap out of it.
     3 I am so sad or unhappy that I can't stand it.

2   0 I am not particularly discouraged about the future.
     1 I feel discouraged about the future.
     2 I feel I have nothing to look forward to.
     3 I feel that the future is hopeless and that things cannot improve.

3   0 I do not feel like a failure.
     1 I feel I have failed more than the average person.
     2 As I look back on my life, all I can see is a lot of failures.
     3 I feel I am a complete failure as a person.

4   0 I get as much satisfaction out of things as I used to.
     1 I don't enjoy things the way I used to.
     2 I don't get real satisfaction out of anything anymore.
     3 I am dissatisfied or bored with everything.

5   0 I don't feel particularly guilty.
     1 I feel guilty a good part of the time.
     2 I feel quite guilty most of the time.
     3 I feel guilty all of the time.

6   0 I don't feel I am being punished.
     1 I feel I may be punished.
     2 I expect to be punished.
     3 I feel I am being punished.

7 0 I don't feel disappointed in myself.
     1 I am disappointed in myself.
     2 I am disgusted with myself.
     3 I hate myself.

8 0 I don't feel I am any worse than anybody else.
     1 I am critical of myself for my weaknesses or mistakes.
     2 I blame myself all the time for my faults.
     3 I blame myself for everything bad that happens.

9 0 I don't have any thoughts of killing myself.
     1 I have thoughts of killing myself, but I would not carry them out.
     2 I would like to kill myself.
     3 I would kill myself if I had the chance.

10 0 I don't cry any more than usual.
     1 I cry more now than I used to.
     2 I cry all the time now.
     3 I used to be able to cry, but now I can't cry even though I want to.

11 0 I am no more irritated now than I ever am.
     1 I get annoyed or irritated more easily than I used to.
     2 I feel irritated all the time now.
     3 I don't get irritated at all by the things that used to irritate me.

12 0 I have not lost interest in other people.
     1 I am less interested in other people than I used to be.
     2 I have lost most of my interest in other people.
     3 I have lost all of my interest in other people.

13 0 I make decisions about as well as I ever could.
     1 I put off making decisions more than I used to.
     2 I have greater difficulty in making decisions than before.
     3 I can't make decisions at all anymore.

14 0 I don't feel I look any worse than I used to.
     1 I am worried that I am looking old or unattractive.
     2 I feel that there are permanent changes in my appearance that make me look
       unattractive.
     3 I believe that I look ugly.

15 0 I can work about as well as before.
     1 It takes an extra effort to get started at doing something.
     2 I have to push myself very hard to do anything.
     3 I can't do any work at all.

16 0 I can sleep as well as usual.
     1 I don't sleep as well as I used to.
     2 I wake up 1–2 hours earlier than usual and find it hard to get back to sleep.
     3 I wake up several hours earlier than I used to and cannot get back to sleep.

17 0 I don't get more tired than usual.
     1 I get tired more easily than I used to.
     2 I get tired from doing almost anything.
     3 I am too tired to do anything.

18   0 My appetite is no worse than usual.
    1 My appetite is not as good as it used to be.
    2 My appetite is much worse now.
    3 I have no appetite at all anymore.

19   0 I haven't lost much weight, if any, lately.
    1 I have lost more than 5 pounds.   I am purposely trying to lose
    2 I have lost more than 10 pounds.   weight by eating less.
    3 I have lost more than 15 pounds.   Yes _____ No _____

20   0 I am no more worried about my health than usual.
    1 I am worried about physical problems such as aches and pains; or upset stomach; or constipation.
    2 I am very worried about physical problems and it's hard to think of much else.
    3 I am so worried about my physical problems that I cannot think about anything else.

21   0 I have not noticed any recent change in my interest in sex.
    1 I am less interested in sex than I used to be.
    2 I am much less interested in sex now.
    3 I have lost interest in sex completely.

What Is Usual
A depressive mood, while not usually normal, can exist in the face of the loss of a loved one (including separation and divorce), loss of one's job, loss of one's social standing, loss of one's health and accompanying money problems. The despondency is usually limited to the situation and its after effects. It is not usual to persist in avoiding pleasure and to brood incessantly. Responses to the Beck Depression Inventory (your score is determined by adding all the circled numbers) should total less than 10.

What You Need
You need a willingness to seek a medical consultation should there be any hint of a "blue" mood. Medical consultation is also warranted if you have noticed that you are having trouble sleeping, that you are always tired, that your appetite is gone, that you are always brooding, that you have become indifferent to people and things, and that life just is not fun anymore. You owe it to yourself to try and uncover any possible organic or physical cause of your depression.

Insofar as the questionnaire goes, honesty in answering, and appropriate medical consultation or attention if indicated, can be the first step toward relief.

What to Watch Out For
- Self-pity, where you enjoy the attention given you while you make others miserable
- Using your depression as an excuse for your failures, misbehavior or inadequacy
- Drugs that can be to blame; check with your doctor or pharmacist.

What the Test Results Can Mean
A score of 10 or more on the Beck Depression Inventory is suggestive of depression and warrants a medical consultation; 16 or more warrants medical attention; and a score of 20 or more warrants immediate medical attention to the point of seeking out an emergency medical facility if a doctor is not instantly available.

REFLEX TESTING

A reflex test is a measure of the body's reaction to stimulation. In effect, it takes into consideration the ability to perceive a stimulus (to the skin, the muscles, the surface of the eye), the efficacy of a nerve to carry recognition of that stimulus to the spinal cord (and sometimes to the brain), the ability of the nervous system to interpret the stimulus, the efficacy of another nerve to carry back a response to that stimulus to the proper organ (usually a muscle) and the ability to respond physically. In other words, a reflex can indicate brain, spinal cord, nerve and muscle well-being, or lack of same.

The most common reflex test is the knee-jerk (Figure 30); tapping the skin over the patellar tendon just below the kneecap (usually with a rubber hammer) stretches the attached thigh muscle, and that muscle normally responds by contracting (shortening), lifting the lower leg and foot up suddenly and involuntarily. Virtually every muscle in the body can be tested this way, but only a few such tests are routinely performed. Besides the patellar, or knee-jerk, reflex, they include:

- The biceps reflex—hold the individual's arm partially flexed, with your thumb over the inside bend at the elbow (just about where blood is usually taken for laboratory testing); at this point your thumb is over the tendon from the biceps (the large upper arm muscle), which lifts the lower arm; a tap on your thumb should cause the person's lower arm to lift
- The wrist reflex—hold the individual's lower arm at the elbow so that the arm is parallel to the floor and the wrist hangs down loosely; tap the upper surface of the lower arm with a rubber hammer about two-thirds of the way down the arm between the elbow and wrist; when the rubber hammer strikes the main muscle attached to the wrist, it causes that muscle to contract, suddenly raising the wrist and hand

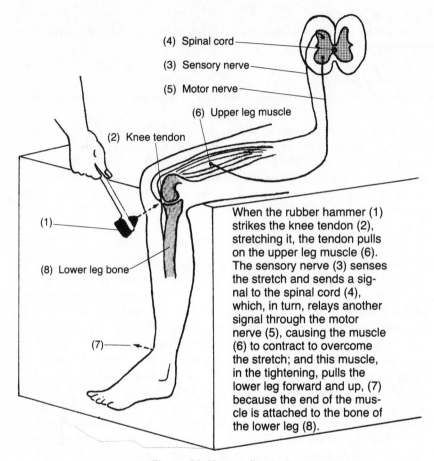

(4) Spinal cord

(3) Sensory nerve

(5) Motor nerve

(6) Upper leg muscle

(2) Knee tendon

(1)

(8) Lower leg bone

(7)

When the rubber hammer (1) strikes the knee tendon (2), stretching it, the tendon pulls on the upper leg muscle (6). The sensory nerve (3) senses the stretch and sends a signal to the spinal cord (4), which, in turn, relays another signal through the motor nerve (5), causing the muscle (6) to contract to overcome the stretch; and this muscle, in the tightening, pulls the lower leg forward and up, (7) because the end of the muscle is attached to the bone of the lower leg (8).

Figure 30. Knee reflex test.

• The ankle-jerk reflex (Achilles reflex)—with one hand holding the individual's foot so that the toes point upward, tap the Achilles tendon (in the center of the back of the foot, just above the heel); this contracts the large muscle in the back of the leg and normally causes the foot to point downward.

The above reflexes are called "deep" reflexes, because the force of a light blow is required to stretch a tendon under the skin. In contrast, there are the "superficial" reflexes, where, to elicit a response, the surface need only be gently touched or stroked. A few of these include:

• The neck-pupil reflex—if you pinch the skin at the back of the neck, it should cause the pupils to dilate (see Eye and Vision Tests, **Pupillary Reflex** tests)

- Corneal reflex—if you touch the surface of the white part of the eye (the cornea), the eyelids should blink
- Abdominal reflexes—a gentle stroke on the skin above, below or to the side of the umbilicus (navel) should cause the muscles under the skin to pull the umbilicus toward the direction of the stroke
- The cremasteric reflex—a gentle stroke on the skin just inside the upper thigh adjacent to the scrotum (the sac that holds the testicle) should cause the scrotum to rise up, on the side that was stroked, toward the abdomen because of the contraction of the cremasteric muscle
- One unusual reflex is called the Babinski test: hold the foot by the ankle and stroke the sole of the foot firmly with a blunt object from heel to toe; usually toes curl and point downward
- The cold face reflex—a large ice bag is placed over the entire face and held there for one minute; normally this causes the pulse rate to slow momentarily (see Heart and Circulation Tests, **Pulse Measurements**) through nerve impulses acting on the parasympathetic nervous system (see Heart and Circulation Tests, **Cold Pressor and Finger Wrinkle** tests).

Muscles to be tested should be relaxed; if they are tense before testing, the normal reaction may not occur. One way to induce relaxation in other muscles is to have the individual hold his or her hands together by the fingers and try to pull them apart; this action usually allows the other muscles to relax.

The value of reflex testing is that it not only offers signs of brain, nerve and/or muscle disease, but it can also give a fairly accurate picture of just where the trouble lies. The more muscles and nerve pathways are tested, the more precise the location of the pathology. Reflex testing usually accompanies tests for touch, feel and temperature discrimination (see Brain and Nervous System Tests, **Sensory Testing**) and can also include **Smell Function** and **Taste Function** tests.

What Is Usual
Reflex reactions should all be present and of a reasonable nature; that is, not too weak, nor too strong or forceful. You will have to observe a few reflex reactions to become familiar with "normal," and it might be best to watch your doctor test your own reflexes and those of others at first to learn the "normal" response. The strength of reflex reactions should be the same on both sides of the body.

What You Need
A rubber percussion hammer can make reflex testing easier; it costs from $1.00 to $3.00. One containing a pin and brush (for sensory testing) costs from $4.00 to $5.00. In most instances, however, the edge of the hand and

the fingers will serve adequately. You will need an ice bag for the cold face reflex test.

What to Watch Out For
Do not hit too hard; in most instances a gentle tap will suffice. Be sure the individual being tested is relaxed. If you do not elicit a reflex reaction at first, be sure you are striking the proper spot. Do not perform the cold face reflex test on someone with known heart disease until you have discussed it with your doctor.

What the Test Results Can Mean
Failure to elicit a reflex reaction with proper technique and relaxed muscles usually indicates a nerve-spinal cord problem; excessive or violent reflex re-actions usually indicate brain involvement. At times deep reflexes will be present, but superficial ones will be absent; the opposite can also happen. The absence or exaggeration of any reflex warrants medical attention; there are innumerable conditions that can cause these abnormal test results, and the earlier the specific cause is detected, the more efficacious is treatment.

A positive Babinski reflex (where the toes curl upward and spread apart) can be an ominous warning of serious brain disease. With the cold face reflex test, failure of the pulse to slow noticeably can be a sign of diabetes, multiple sclerosis or even the consequence of a little stroke that might have gone un-detected. Obviously, any doubt about the results of these reflex tests warrants medical attention.

As an incidental observation, many doctors feel that a slow or seemingly momentarily delayed ankle-jerk (Achilles) reflex is a reasonable sign of thy-roid disease. On the other hand, if repeated testing of the ankle-jerk reflex seems to show an increasing time delay before responding, after an initial normal response, it can be a reasonable sign of diabetes. Either observation warrants medical attention.

SENSORY

There are many different tests that help measure your ability to perceive various sensations (pain discrimination and pressure as opposed to light touch, differences in temperature, tuning fork vibrations, position sense and the ability to recognize form and writing when applied to the skin). When these tests are performed along with **Reflex Testing**, they can help diagnose brain, nerve and spinal cord problems. Because a doctor knows just where each nerve functions anatomically, it is usually possible to pinpoint the exact loca-tion of the pathology. These tests also help explain some of the many "sensations" some people complain of: burning, tingling, pins and needles, unexplained pain or the absence of any feeling at all (numbness). And sensory testing can be quite valuable in detecting malingerers.

The following sensory tests are performed with the individual's eyes closed or blindfolded, so that the measurements are more objective; they are usually performed all over the body surfaces and extremities:

- Pinprick—it is usual for an individual to feel the pain of a slight pinprick on the body, and it should feel the same all over; at the same time, the individual should be able to discriminate between a pinprick and the push of a pencil eraser
- Light touch discrimination—an individual should be able to discern the difference between the touch of a piece of cotton, a small brush, the light stroke of a fingertip, and between coarse cotton and silk
- Temperature discrimination—when two tubes of water, one warm and the other cool, are individually placed against the skin, a person should easily be able to tell the difference
- Tuning fork—when the base of a vibrating tuning fork is placed on a bony surface (elbow, ankle, spine), an individual should be able to feel the vibrations for as long as the examiner can
- Position sense—an individual should be able to tell when his or her thumb, fingers and big toe have been pointed up or down
- Distance discrimination—when two pins or other objects are placed near each other on the skin, an individual should be able to tell about how far apart they are
- Stereognosis—an individual should be able to recognize and describe the shape of a solid object (coin, button, marble, pencil stub) placed in the hand
- Small-corks—this test is best performed on another family member rather than one's self; obtain four small corks of different sizes ranging from one-half inch to one and one-quarter inches in size, each varying by one-quarter inch; after placing them first in one hand and then the other of a blindfolded person ask that person—using that one hand and its fingers only—to tell how many corks there are and then to hand them back according to size starting with the largest one (if a cork drops, place it back in the subject's hand and continue with the size discrimination)
- Graphesthesia—an individual should be able to recognize and describe a large letter or numeral traced by the examiner's finger or a pencil on the palm of the hand, the abdomen and the leg.

These sensory tests are but a very few that can be performed, but they are sufficient to help signal some early warning signs of disease or hysteria.

What Is Usual
"Normal" responses are noted in each test description.

What You Need
Other than the tuning fork (the same one used in **Hearing Function** tests), which costs from $8.00 to $10.00, most other test equipment can be found around the home. Small jars may be used in place of the test tubes. Corks are available at hardware stores.

What to Watch Out For
Be sure the individual being examined keeps his or her eyes closed at all times; there is a great temptation to "peek," and this, of course, nullifies any test observation. Keep a careful record of your findings; then, when you repeat the same test in the same location, you can tell if there are changes or if the individual was trying to mislead you. Some examiners use a washable fabric marker to identify the skin areas tested for exact repeat testing a short time later.

What the Test Results Can Mean
An abnormal result (failure to perceive what "normal" people can feel and interpret) can be caused by so many different conditions—from disease to dietary deficiencies—that it would be impossible to list them; suffice it to say that any lack of sensory function warrants medical consultation. It takes a physician, with years of experience, to be able to discern the exact anatomical distribution of each nerve on the skin's surface (called a dermatome). For example, if the complaint is one of numbness in the knee, the doctor will determine whether that numbness follows the expected nerve distribution; if it does not, it is just as important to seek the reason for the pretense, which may be hysteria (severe emotional upset) or malingering. An inability to discern the number of corks in one's hand or to be unable to pass them back in proper order according to size can be a sign of a nerve disorder and warrants medical attention.

SMELL FUNCTION

If you think testing for the ability to smell normally seems superfluous, then you are not aware of the constant jeopardy in which millions of people live because they cannot detect dangerous chemical fumes, escaping gas from a stove or heater, smoke from a fire, or the odor of spoiled or contaminated food.

In some instances, the sense of smell is a combination of both smell and taste (see Brain and Nervous System Tests, **Taste Function** testing). Smell

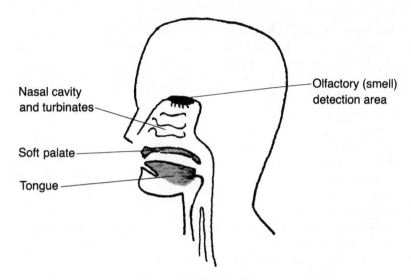

Figure 31. Smell function.

function ability, called olfaction, varies greatly among people: Some are unable to smell anything at all, called anosmia; some have a decreased ability to smell, called hyposmia; some have perversions of odors, called dysosmia; and others can be extra-sensitive to odors to the point of constant discomfort. Pregnant women are often hypersensitive to odors.

Because odors are not recognized until they reach the olfactory nerve endings in the uppermost part of the nasal cavity (at or above eye level) (Figure 31), it becomes obvious why someone with sinus problems (see Miscellaneous Tests, **Sinus Transillumination** test), a cold or hay fever can have smell impairment at times and then have normal smell function at other times. Smell function should be tested for whenever there is a loss of appetite and diminished enjoyment of food; if there is no obvious allergy or infection affecting the nose, it could be an early warning sign of brain or nerve disease. A sudden aversion to certain food odors usually considered pleasant (chocolate, roast beef, fresh-brewed coffee) can be one of the first signs of cancer somewhere in the body. Decreased smell function is found in several other diseases.

Some drugs can reduce or temporarily eliminate smell function; cocaine inhaled through the nose can also act as an anesthetic on the olfactory nerves; the excessive use of nose drops and drugs used to treat thyroid disease causes anosmia; and, certain antibiotics can have a side effect in which the ability to detect or differentiate odors is reduced.

Exposure to toxic heavy metals, industrial chemicals and dusts also can diminish the sense of smell.

What is Usual

With the nasal passages clear, and pressure placed against one of the nostrils to close that side, you should be able to detect and discern different odors—especially familiar ones—through the open side of the nose with the eyes closed. Both sides should detect smells equally. The most common aromas used to test smell function include:

- Onion or garlic
- Chocolate
- Mint (fresh-picked leaves)
- Instant coffee
- Turpentine
- Perfume (or fresh flowers)
- Fresh tobacco (usually pipe tobacco, both before and while smoking)
- A burning paper match (or burning paper in an ashtray), usually performed as the last test because of its possible irritating effect.

Do not try to smell ammonia or menthol; they can irritate the nose and give a false-positive reaction that seems to be smell but is not indicative of smell function.

What You Need

At least three of the above-listed items are required. Ideally, with the exception of the burning match, they should be in a tightly closed container until opened for two to three seconds. For very precise testing, you can construct a modified Elsberg apparatus (Figure 32), using a glass jar with a two-holed rubber stopper allowing glass or plastic tubing to be inserted into the jar. Insert the tube gently into one nostril; then close off the opposite nostril and breathe in. The jar, tubings and stopper can be obtained at any scientific equipment store for less than $1.00. If one or both sides of the nose seem obstructed due to a cold or allergy, you might want to drop or spray a nasal decongestant into the nose about a half-hour prior to testing.

What to Watch Out For

If you are testing someone else, occasionally substitute plain water as a test material; it should have no odor and can help eliminate subjective or hallucinatory responses. If nasal decongestants do not open the nasal passageways within 30 minutes, do not repeat their use; put off the testing for another day. It is a good idea to test smell function prior to undergoing any nose operation (rhinoplasty); in that way you will always be aware of any loss of smell as a consequence of surgery.

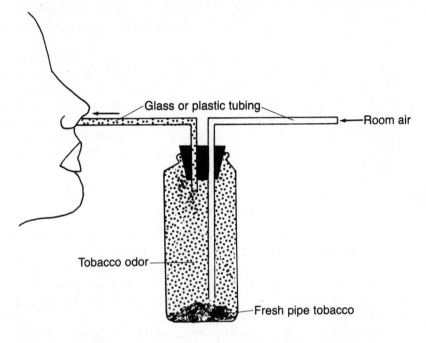

Glass or plastic tubing

Room air

Tobacco odor

Fresh pipe tobacco

Figure 32. Testing smell function using modified Elsberg apparatus.

What the Test Results Can Mean

Any noticeable loss of smell function, not related to temporarily blocked nasal passages, especially if olfaction was previously thought to be "normal," can point to several different diseases. In addition to brain pathology or nerve disease, it could be the consequence of a circulatory problem, such as a little stroke. This is even more likely if smell function is diminished or lost on only one side of the nose; a medical consultation is warranted. Thyroid disease, infections such as encephalitis, pneumonia, many lung conditions, multiple sclerosis, head injuries, nutritional problems and, of course, cancer can also cause interference with the ability to detect odors. A sudden noticing of "foul" odors when no one else perceives them can be the first indication of depression or a neurosis (see Breath and Lung Tests, **Breath Odor and Sputum** tests). A loss of smell and taste can also be attributed to a dietary deficiency of zinc. And about one out of every five people with a decreased sense of smell ends up with a diagnosis of idiopathic (meaning the cause cannot be determined) anosmia. Absent or unusual smell function warrants a medical consultation, if for no other reason than to rule out any underlying problem. If nothing else, testing smell function will let you know if you are able perceive odoriferous warnings of possible dangers. If you find you are unable to notice smoke, it would be advisable to install smoke detectors throughout your residence.

Note: When the 1982 cyanide adulterated Extra-Strength Tylenol capsule tragedy occurred in Chicago, it had been believed that most people could easily smell the so-called bitter almond odor of that deadly poison which had been mixed into the capsules. Further investigation revealed that more than half of all lay persons and most doctors in the Medical Examiner's Office were unable to detect cyanide's characteristic odor. Now pathologists are tested for their ability to smell the poison and, if unable to do so, must work with an assistant who is able to recognize a cyanide odor.

TASTE FUNCTION

The sense of taste is actually a combination of taste and smell (see Brain and Nervous System Tests, **Smell Function** testing). Having a stuffy nose can diminish the sense of taste. It has always been believed that it was the primary function of the tongue to distinguish saltiness, sweetness, sourness and bitterness, but in addition to the tongue, taste buds have been found on the palate, pharynx, epiglottis, tonsils and even the mucosa of the lips and cheeks. Loss or diminution of taste and smell can be caused by many factors, from ordinary colds to cancer. It is now believed that a loss of taste or changes in the sense of taste can be an early sign of cancer; the taste changes reduce the desire to eat, causing weight loss once thought to be from the cancer itself. It has been estimated that more than 2 million Americans suffer some loss of taste and/or smell.

Total loss of taste function is called ageusia; decreased sensitivity to taste or partial loss of taste is called hypogeusia. Hallucinations of taste, called phantogeusia, and distorted taste, called dysgeusia, can occur normally during pregnancy. Many drugs can cause any or all of these problems; some include antifungus preparations, antibiotics, medicines to treat arthritis and muscle pains, Parkinson's disease, thyroid disease and vaginitis, to name but a few. Even toothpaste that contains sodium lauryl sulfate (see the list of ingredients on the label) can cause interference with taste function.

Older people sometimes seem to have a slightly decreased sensitivity to salt and bitter flavors and will often require extra amounts of salt to make foods taste "right." A number of nutritional deficiencies, especially a lack of zinc in the diet, are also related to taste impairment; saliva must contain a zinc-protein compound to allow normal taste function.

What Is Usual

Different areas of the tongue are sensitive to different tastes. The four taste groups and their primary areas are (Figure 33):

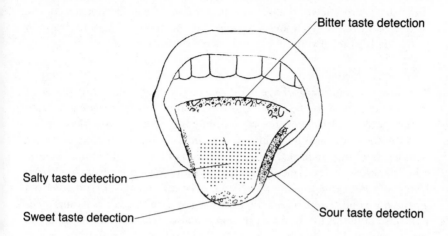

Figure 33. Areas of the tongue involved in tasting selectivity.

* Bitter—at the back of the tongue
* Salty—on the upper surface, toward the front
* Sour—at the edges on either side
* Sweet—at the tip.

If you place a drop of an applicable sample solution on the appropriate area of the tongue, you should be able to distinguish each one distinctly; as a control, there should be no taste perception if a drop of distilled water is used in place of a solution. It is also possible for taste sensations to be noticed when a drop of sample solution is placed in other than the appropriate area, but initially the drop should not seem to have as strong a flavor.

What You Need
The test requires an eyedropper and some distilled water to use as a control and to make up applicable solutions:

* Bitter—quinine water, undiluted
* Salty—one teaspoon of salt dissolved in four ounces of distilled water
* Sour—one teaspoon of vinegar dissolved in one ounce of distilled water
* Sweet—one teaspoon of sugar dissolved in four ounces of distilled water.

What to Watch Out For
Do not attempt taste function testing if you have a cold, sinusitis or simply a stuffy nose or if you have recently had alcoholic beverages or been smoking.

Check with your doctor or pharmacist if you are taking medications; find out if the drugs are known to alter taste perception. If you are not sure of the results, blindfold yourself and have someone else place the various drops on your tongue to see if you can correctly perceive the flavors.

What the Test Results can Mean

The most common cause of ageusia is Bell's palsy (an inflammation of one of the main nerves of the face), but this condition makes itself evident because of the paralysis of the face muscles on one side. Other causes of partial or total taste loss, or taste hallucinations, include: brain, nerve, lung and liver diseases; migraine; diabetes; fungus infections of the mouth; tooth troubles; a deficiency of dietary zinc (excess fiber in the diet can prevent zinc from being absorbed from the intestines); and, of course, mental aberrations from a psychotic condition. Decrease in or absence of taste function warrants medical consultation. A loss of taste function can also mean a loss of the ability to avoid toxic substances such as spoiled food or dangerous chemicals that might otherwise have been detected before damage occurred.

GASTROINTESTINAL SYSTEM TESTS

FECES OBSERVATIONS

Although some people find it disturbing simply to look at a bowel movement, the observation of feces (or stool as it is sometimes called) can be one of the simplest, yet best sources of health information, second only to urine testing. Feces, like urine, are a waste product and primarily reflect digestion as opposed to metabolism; normally they consist of food material that could not be digested, some remnants of bile from the liver, intestinal secretions and bacteria. Abnormal constitutents such as blood, foul odor or the absence of certain pigments can be the first clue to pathology and, when detected early enough in the course of disease, can lead to simple, efficient treatment.

Most people on a typical diet produce approximately 100 to 300 grams (from 3 to 10 ounces) of feces a day, of which close to 70 percent is water. The rest is about two-thirds fiber (cellulose, the skin and seeds of fruits and vegetables) and one-third normal intestinal bacteria, which are supposed to be present. Home tests on feces include: observation of color and consistency, odor, whether the feces float in the water or sink to the bottom of the bowl; whether or not blood, white blood cells (leukocytes) or glucose are present; the degree of acidity; and indirectly, the search for pinworms and other parasites.

What Is Usual
Although most people have a bowel movement daily, more than one a day or only one every two or three days may not be abnormal; if the amount remains reasonably related to the diet (large quantities of fruits, vegetables and whole grains tend to increase the amount of feces, while proteins and liquids tend to decrease it), little attention need be paid to feces volume. The color should be from medium to dark brown and homogeneous (of uniform color) throughout, but again, diet and drugs must be considered: Eating large amounts of green vegetables can give feces a greenish hue, and some antibiotics can cause feces to have a yellowish tinge. Food coloring or dyes in drugs can also alter stool color. The consistency should be firm, but not hard or watery; each segment should be from one-half inch to one inch in diame-

ter. A diet high in fiber will usually cause the feces to float. The odor, while never described as pleasant, should not be too obtrusive. The pH should be close to neutral (7); large amounts of meat in the diet can make it more alkaline (7–8.5), while large quanities of carbohydrates make it more acid (6–7). There should be little or no glucose and no evidence of blood, white blood cells or parasites. Eating rare meats, certain vegetables, fruits and vigorous brushing of the teeth are a few of the things that can cause a false-positive blood test.

What You Need

A willingness to study a feces sample is required.

You should obtain one of the many test kits available to detect occult blood (occult meaning blood is present but not visible to the naked eye). Most doctors will give you, usually without charge, from one to three kits for feces occult blood testing. Otherwise, there is:

- ColoScreen (available either as a single test or in a package of three plus a positive and negative standard control check); a box of 100 single or 34 three-test kits costs $27.50
- Hema-Chek; a box of 100 single tests costs $31.00
- Hematest tablets—probably the most sensitive of all the tests to detect occult blood; however, their extreme sensitivity can cause a four-fold increase in false-positive reactions; the tablets come with special filter papers upon which a small portion of the feces specimen is placed; the tablet is then placed on the specimen and a drop or two of water is then applied to the tablet; this test can also be performed following a prostate observation, (see Genitourinary System Tests) by wiping the gloved finger with the Hematest filter paper and placing the tablet on the feces residue that had adhered to the glove. They cost $13.80 for 100 tablets
- Hemoccult II, which comes in sets of three tests and costs $35.00 for 100 three-test kits.

Note: Some of the preceeding tests come with a "developer"—a liquid chemical to complete the detection process; others, for people who just cannot bring themselves to face their feces, may require you to bring the feces specimen to the doctor's office, laboratory or hospital for "developing." Be sure to check whether your occult blood test comes with all the supplies you need.

- Chemstrip 3 or Combistix (also includes glucose and pH testing), which costs from $17.00 to $20.00 for 100 dipsticks
- Chemstrip 5L (includes all the tests in Chemstrip 3 and Combistix plus the test for white blood cells, or leukocytes), which costs about $23.00

per 100 dipsticks, or Chemstrip L (white blood cell test only), which costs $8.00 per 100 dipsticks.

A pocket-sized microscope, such as the Panasonic 30-power light scope, which costs from $20.00 to $30.00, can be used to identify pinworms and some other worm eggs (ova) or segments of parasites such as tapeworms. A few drops of normal or physiological saline (salt solution) are needed to dilute the bit of feces for microscopic examination; it costs about 60 to 75 cents for a one-ounce bottle.

A bedpan or very wide-mouthed, dry, clean jar is needed to collect a feces specimen for testing for pH, glucose, white blood cells and parasites. Unlike tests for occult blood, for these tests to be performed, the feces should not come in contact with toilet paper, urine or water.

It is best to take two samples for testing—one from the surface of the stool segment to detect possible lower bowel bleeding and one from the center to detect possible upper intestinal bleeding.

What to Watch Out For
Follow the directions supplied with each occult blood test kit carefully; one company's kit may vary from that of another company in test procedure. Although you should not eat red meat, radishes, horseradish, broccoli, artichoke, raw mushrooms, cantaloupe or turnips; take aspirin or aspirin-containing products, vitamin C, iron pills or tonics, or cortisone drugs; or brush your teeth for three days prior to testing for occult blood (the test is sensitive enough to detect a trace of blood inadvertently swallowed from gums bruised by vigorous brushing), many doctors require these restrictions for repeat testing only if the first test is positive. Do not test feces from a toilet bowl that contains any chemical bowl cleaner. Should the feces specimen be very dry, place a drop of water on the area of the specimen to be tested and wait 30 seconds before testing.

What the Test Results Can Mean
If feces seem very light brown, gray or even appear to be without color, and you have not been limiting your diet to unusually large amounts of milk, medical attention is warranted; this can mean liver or gallbladder trouble. If there is any red color of the feces not related to eating beets, it could mean rectal bleeding and certainly warrants medical attention. Black or tarry-colored stools not related to large doses of iron must be considered as suspicious evidence of bleeding in the upper portions of the gastrointestinal tract (esophagus, stomach and small intestines); while it could be the consequence of taking large amounts of aspirin, it could also mean some serious gastrointestinal condition, and it warrants medical attention. Greenish colored feces can accompany diarrhea but are not specific for any one condition. A silver

or aluminum colored feces, especially if accompanied by jaundice, could come from a growth blocking the pancreas gland duct and warrants medical attention.

If the consistency of the feces seems to change, particularly if the diameter seems to be much smaller, medical attention is warranted, since this is one of the first signs of an obstructed bowel. Repeated watery feces, especially if mucus is seen, can mean a chronic irritable bowel or an infection by bacteria or parasites such as amebiasis, giardiasis (Figure 34) or typhoid—especially if you have recently been camping out or traveling away from home (see Gastrointestinal System Tests, **String Test**). Infections or parasitic infestations are usually accompanied by feces with a very foul odor, and feces with such an odor should make one think of giardiasis. Repeated episodes of very hard, dry feces mean constipation, most often from a faulty diet, but they could also result from disease, especially in young children, and warrant a medical consultation.

A positive occult blood test after three days of careful dietary, drug, vitamin and tooth care restrictions warrants medical attention; it does not, however, automatically mean cancer. Other conditions such as diverticulitis, hookworms, polyps and simple internal hemorrhoids may be the cause and are usually easily treated. Repeated negative tests in the presence of any bowel discomfort or symptoms do not rule out bowel disease; they warrant a medical consultation.

If there is a suspicion that drinking milk is causing problems (see Gastrointestinal System Tests, **Milk Products (Lactose) Intolerance** test), insert a dipstick into the feces sample to test for pH and glucose, wait 10 seconds, rinse the dipstick and then compare the colors on the container to see whether the feces are very acid (5–6) and glucose is present (it should not be); this helps confirm intolerance to the milk sugar lactose.

The white blood cell (leukocyte) test is usually performed when there are chronic intestinal problems, most often with repeated bouts of diarrhea, frequently showing mucus along with lower bowel cramping. When a dipstick that tests for white blood cells is inserted into a feces specimen for 10 seconds and then rinsed off, a positive test (indicating white blood cells are present) can mean a parasitic infestation, typhoid fever or some other salmonella-type infection, or it can indicate ulcerative colitis. A negative white blood cell test suggests giardiasis, a virus infection or cholera. But then, this much chronic bowel trouble should already have prompted a medical consultation.

When children are persistently scratching their buttocks, and usually the nose as well, think of pinworms as a possible cause; they are the most common of worm infestations. Pinworm infestation often imitates appendicitis in children. Wind a piece of Scotch Tape around the eraser end of a pencil, sticky side out, and during the night touch the sticky surface to and around the anal area of the child (the worms come out at night to lay their eggs after the child has been under a blanket and warmed the buttocks). Spread the Scotch Tape out on a glass slide and search for the eggs (Figure 34) through a pocket microscope; they are quite distinctive. You may have to repeat this test for several nights before the pinworm eggs are detected. If the eggs are seen, a medical consultation is warranted. One dose of a medicine (to be taken by everyone in the family at the same time) can easily cure the condition. Other parasite egg-looking objects and even some worm segments may sometimes be seen on the Scotch Tape or when a piece of feces about the size of a match head is placed on a glass slide and mixed with two or three drops of normal saline; a feces sample is more apt to show evidence of worms if it is taken from the surface of either end of the segment or adjacent to a speck of mucus.

Tapeworms (Figure 34) can come from eating raw or inadequately cooked meat (steak tartare), raw fish (sashimi or some sushi preparations) or by unconsciously tasting raw food during preparation (such as when making gefilte fish). Hookworm infestation (Figure 34) and strongyloidiasis (a form of roundworm) (Figure 34) can come from going barefoot on ground (or pavement) where dogs have deposited excrement containing worms or where bird droppings are found; the worms burrow through the skin of the feet to enter the body. Both of these worms can cause skin lesions, but hookworms also cause anemia (see Blood Tests, **Hemoglobin** test), while strongyloidiasis can cause a cough and other symptoms similar to asthma. Any suggestion of parasites in the feces warrants a medical consultation.

MILK PRODUCTS (LACTOSE) INTOLERANCE

Most milk products contain lactose, a form of sugar, which requires an enzyme, lactase, to metabolize it. Some people do not naturally produce sufficient lactase to break down the ingested milk sugar adequately, and as a result, they may suffer uncomfortable symptoms after drinking milk or eating foods containing milk products, such as ice cream, commercially prepared bakery products, desserts, soups, frozen fruits and vegetables, baby foods, yogurt and foods where "milk solids," "caseinates" or "whey" appears on the label. Some other commercial products such as instant coffee; powdered beverages; breaded foods; hot dogs; bologna; canned fruits and vegetables; cookie, cake and pancake mix; candies; and prepared sauces can also contain lactose as an ingredient, but it may not appear on the label. Soft cheeses also contain lactose, but the sugar is usually broken down and disappears in the making of hard cheese. And lactose is commonly used as a binder in the manufacture of medicine tablets and vitamin pills.

Figure 34. Parasites, or their eggs, that can cause intestinal diseases. The six illustrations are as they might be observed through a 30-power pocket light microscope. All but the *Giardia* can sometimes be seen with the naked eye.

Giardia lamblia, the cause of giardiasis.

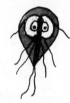

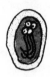

Trophozoite
(live, active phase)

Cyst
(inactive, resting phase)

-Less than 1 mm-

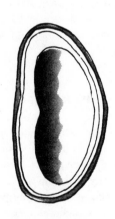

Approximately 2 mm

Pinworm egg
(*Enterobius vermicularis*)

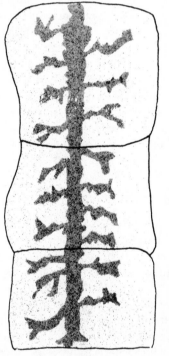

From ½ to 2 inches or 10 to 50 mm

Three connected segments of *Taenia solium*, the pork tapeworm. Beef and fish tapeworms are similar in appearance. The entire pork tapeworm is from 6 to 12 feet long; a beef tapeworm is from 12 to 35 feet; and a fish tapeworm from 10 to 40 feet. All can be composed of hundreds of segments.

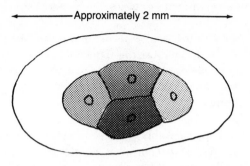

Hookworm egg
(*Necator americanus*)

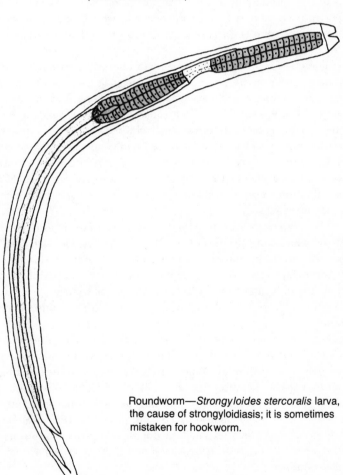

Roundworm—*Strongyloides stercoralis* larva,
the cause of strongyloidiasis; it is sometimes
mistaken for hookworm.

The most common symptoms of lactose intolerance include:

- Bloating and flatulence—excessive and uncomfortable amounts of gas in the abdomen, which can cause the abdomen to swell
- Borborygmi—rumbling abdominal noises
- Diarrhea
- Intestinal cramps.

All these symptoms appear within 30 to 90 minutes after the ingestion of a full glass of whole milk or the equivalent in milk products; some people can tolerate a very small amount of lactose (a teaspoon of cream in their coffee), so the quantity of milk products must also be taken into account. If you happen to be of Mediterranean origin, are Arab, black, Oriental or of Ashkenazi Jewish (Central and Eastern European) ancestry, your chances of suffering from lactose intolerance are much greater than if your forebears came from Northern Europe.

The essence of the problem seems to be that individuals with insufficient lactase cannot break down the milk sugar, lactose, into more simple sugar molecules (glucose and galactose), and therefore, it cannot be properly digested. Undigested lactose then causes excess body fluids to be drawn into the upper portion of the intestines, and when the heavily watered food moves through the bowel, it causes increased acidity and an increased amount of gas along with a watery bowel movement. Milk product intolerance is not the same as milk allergy (see Miscellaneous Tests, **Allergy Patch Testing and Elimination Diet**); it rarely causes a rash or other skin manifestations of hypersensitivity.

The simplest way to test for lactose intolerance is to eliminate as many lactose-containing products from the diet as possible. If formerly frequent gastrointestinal symptoms disappear or even lessen considerably within two to three days, this is the first step; the second step is to drink a glass of whole milk (use only one-quarter glass of milk for children) and wait to see if bloating or cramps recur, followed by a bout of diarrhea within the next 12 to 24 hours.

A more definitive test, if drinking milk does cause symptoms, is to add LactAid, a commercial preparation of lactase, to the milk and again wait to see if symptoms develop. When discomfort occurs after drinking milk without LactAid but not after drinking milk with LactAid, this should confirm the condition, and the treatment is to eliminate lactose-containing products where possible and to make LactAid part of your diet where lactose cannot be avoided.

Other confirmatory tests include the use of dipstick-type testing for pH and glucose (see Blood Tests, **Glucose** test and Gastrointestinal System Tests, **Feces Observations**).

What Is Usual

While most people have no trouble drinking and digesting milk and milk products, it is believed that more than 10 percent of Americans have an inability to digest lactose. Again, the intolerance to lactose in milk can also be one of degree; some people have no uncomfortable symptoms until they exceed a certain quantity of the milk sugar.

What You Need

A willingness to try to identify foods containing lactose and the desire to avoid those foods are required, as is a small quantity of LactAid. A supply sufficient to "treat" 12 quarts of milk costs from $2.75 to $3.00 and is available without a prescription. In some parts of the country, dairies offer milk already treated with LactAid. Should you wish to perform blood and feces tests, you will need appropriate dipsticks, described under each test.

What to Watch Out For

Do not attempt the test if you have any sort of intestinal infection or upset, if you have undergone surgery or X-rays of your abdomen within the past two months or if you are taking antibiotics, especially penicillin or neomycin; these interferences, while not harmful, tend to give temporary false-positive reactions.

If you do avoid lactose-containing foods, be sure to supplement your diet with other foods containing calcium (hard cheese, green leafy vegetables, sardines, etc.) and vitamin D.

If you have diabetes, do not use LactAid until you talk with your physician; it can add a bit more glucose to your system.

What the Test Results Can Mean

Avoidance of milk and milk products containing lactose along with relief of gastrointestinal discomfort is a result sufficient unto itself. The use of LactAid can prevent your having to eliminate many favorite foods from your diet. If avoidance of lactose or the use of LactAid does not give obvious relief, there is always the rare possibility that the gastrointestinal symptoms are caused by allergy (see Miscellaneous Tests, **Allergy Patch Testing** and **Elimination Diet**). Should nothing seem to help, a medical consultation is warranted; other conditions that can imitate milk product intolerance include: thyroid disease, Crohn's disease (an inflammation of the lower part of the small intestines), sprue (a malabsorption problem) and kwashiorkor (primarily a protein deficiency that can cause mental irritation and apathy in addition to symptoms resembling those of lactose intolerance).

MOUTH AND THROAT OBSERVATIONS

It is as much of a medical test to search for abnormalities in and on the body as it is to detect the presence of some abnormal substance in blood or urine. To examine the inside of the mouth and notice the sudden presence of a new white spot that will not wipe away could be a most valuable test result, especially if it turns out to be an early enough sign of cancer to allow simple, effective treatment. Nearly 20 percent of mouth cancers start out as a white patch, or leukoplakia. On the other hand, similar-looking white patches could also be lichen planus, a disease with no known cause that does not require specific treatment, other than symptomatic relief of any irritation. White patches in the mouth could also mean thrush (candidiasis or moniliasis), a fungus infection that commonly comes about while taking antibiotics or cortisone drugs, or they might also signal diabetes or leukemia. It is not that you can be expected to specifically diagnose unusual mouth lesions, but if you regularly search the mouth and throat areas so that you become aware of what they usually look like, you can then notice an unusual lesion almost as soon as it appears. And when it comes to tests for tumors and other illnesses that can reveal themselves through mouth and throat manifestations, observation alone can far outdo the most sophisticated chemical analysis or X-ray.

Start by inspecting the lips; blisterlike lesions most often are herpes (see Miscellaneous Tests, **Skin Observations**), but also look for any irregularities, cracking, drying or dark blue patches on the lip surfaces. Next, using a bright flashlight and, if necessary, a wooden tongue depressor (Figure 35), look at the gums and then at and under the tongue. Then inspect the insides of the cheeks. Continue your visual observation over the palate (roof of the mouth) and then back toward the throat, comparing both sides where the tonsils are (or were); also note the color and size of the uvula (the small flap of tissue that hangs down from the middle of the top of the back of the mouth; it looks somewhat like a tonsil). Finally, survey the back of the throat (the pharynx), looking particularly for redness, any mucus drippings, sores or a membrane (a thin film that seems to be covering the throat). After observation comes palpation. Slowly but firmly slide your fingers over the top and under the tongue and then sweep it over the inner cheek surfaces; see if you can feel any small bump or irregularity, even when nothing is evident to the eye. The simple secret of effective mouth and throat observation is to learn by practicing on an individual who has no fever, no mouth complaints or symptoms, and no sore throat.

What Is Usual
The lips should be moist and without any lesions or discoloration. The gums should be uniformly pink and show no signs of bleeding. The tongue and the

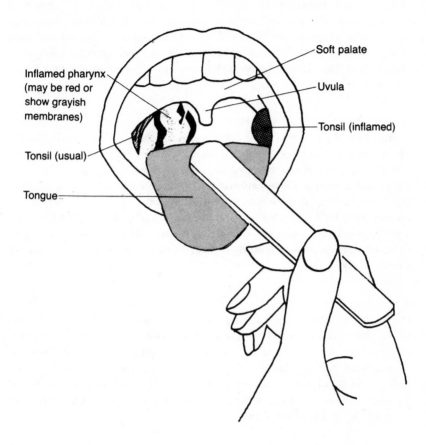

Soft palate

Inflamed pharynx
(may be red or
show grayish
membranes)

Uvula

Tonsil (inflamed)

Tonsil (usual)

Tongue

Figure 35. Mouth and throat observations.

Note: The adenoids (tonsillar tissue) are usually not seen, as they lie behind and
above the soft palate.

inside of the mouth should be smooth, with no bumps or plaques (small flat
patches) either seen or felt. When the tongue is protruded (stuck out), it
should come out straight and not lean toward one side or the other. On some
people the tongue will show furrows (little valleys) crossways (from side to
side), or it may show patches of red, brighter than the rest of the tongue
(called geographic tongue, because it almost looks like a relief map); these
manifestations are usually inherited and are probably normal. The tonsils, if

still present, should be of equal size, pink and have thin grooves running up and down; sometimes tonsils, even though present, are difficult to see in their natural pockets. After a tonsillectomy, the pockets where they once were should be hollowed out, pink and smooth. The uvula should be small, pink and hang straight down. The back of the throat should look evenly pink over the entire surface, and there should be no evidence of any mucus dripping down from the nasal cavity.

What You Need

A bright flashlight and some tongue depressors (also called tongue blades), which come in two sizes: adult and children's; they cost $3.00 for a box of 100. If you have an otoscope (see Ear Observations and Hearing Tests, **Ear Canal and Eardrum Observations**), it may have come with an attachment that holds a tongue depressor in place just under the light bulb. If not, special tongue blade light sets (one is called Oralume) are available at $15.00. The Sears Roebuck Orotoscope, which includes an otoscope, also has a fiber optic-lighted tongue depressor (you do not need the wooden tongue depressors); it costs $17.00.

What to Watch Out For

Do not use a spoon or something similar in place of a tongue depressor; sudden biting down could chip a tooth. If it is difficult to see the back of the throat, grasp the tip of the tongue with a dry gauze pad; it will keep the tongue from slipping. If the individual being examined tends to gag when saying "aaaah" or while you are trying to see the back of the mouth and throat, tell the person to stick out his or her tongue and pant like a dog; this can help eliminate the gag reflex.

What the Test Results Can Mean

Any obvious lesion on the lips or in the mouth or throat, especially the sudden appearance of a new, pigmented one that does not go away after a few days, warrants a medical consultation. Even herpes–like lesions (unless they have been recurring almost all your life) warrant a medical consultation to be sure the disease is limited to the mouth. Dark blue dots over the lips could be a sign of an intestinal disorder and warrant a medical consultation. Bleeding gums most often come from overzealous brushing of the teeth, but they may also come from poor tooth care (see Miscellaneous Tests, **Dental Plaque Disclosure**). Unfortunately, bleeding gums can also be the first sign of blood disorders (especially bleeding tendencies; see Heart and Circulation Tests, **Capillary Fragility** test), leukemia, infections (especially trench mouth), toxic metal poisoning (see Miscellaneous Tests, **Hair Observation and Mineral**

Analysis) and insufficient vitamin C in the diet (see Miscellaneous Tests, **Vitamin C Body Level**). Certain drugs such as Dilantin can cause swollen, bleeding gums, and at times toxic metal poisoning will show itself by a thin, dark line adjacent to the gum line.

If you should feel a lump while rubbing the tongue and cheeks with your finger, it could be a calcified stone in one of the salivary glands, most commonly under the tongue, but these usually pass out with time; if, however, there is any discomfort or any nodule (hard lump), no matter how small, it warrants medical consultation. If the tongue has a smooth, glossy surface or appears unusually dry (without thirst), these could be signs of various anemias or vitamin deficiencies; furrows that run only from front to back could mean an infection, such as syphilis; a hairy tongue (looks dark and furry at the back surface) usually comes from a fungus infection and can occur while taking antibiotic drugs. If the tongue seems larger than usual, it could come from a hormone disorder, an infection, toxic metal poisoning or blocked veins (varicose veins under the tongue are not unusual after 60 years of age). A burning sensation of the tongue may come from smoking, and it seems to be quite common in women during the menopause; it can also come from toxic metal poisoning. Observation of any deviations from what is usual warrants a medical consultation.

If one or both tonsils look enlarged (the grooves disappear), look fiery red or have yellow or white dots over them, they are probably infected. Because tonsillitis could easily turn into an abscess, it warrants immediate medical attention. Any other swelling, especially if seen in only one tonsil, warrants medical consultation. If the uvula is red and swollen, it is more apt to be from an allergic reaction; it should return to normal color and size as the allergy is controlled. If, however, it swells to the point where it could interfere with breathing or swallowing, immediate medical attention is warranted.

A red throat (redder than usual) means some sort of throat infection (pharyngitis); very bright shiny red usually accompanies a streptococcus infection (see Blood Tests, **Streptozyme** test), while a dull red usually accompanies a virus infection or could be from infectious mononucleosis (see Blood Tests, **Mononucleosis** test). If there seems to be a pale membrane or film over the reddened throat, it could mean diphtheria—even in today's world, where all children should have been immunized against this disease. A membrane or film could also be a sign of trench mouth, or Vincent's angina (a severe mouth infection), especially if other areas of the mouth seem to have spots of membrane. Any suspicion of a membrane warrants immediate medical attention. Since a red-looking throat without fever or other symptoms can come from gonorrhea, any red throat that lasts more than one day warrants a medical consultation; if fever occurs and goes above 102° F(38.9C), immediate medical attention is warranted.

STRING TEST

It has been reported in the medical literature that at least 10 percent of the population suffer from heartburn (sometimes called pyrosis), a burning sensation in the chest just behind the sternum, or breastbone. This painful, aching discomfort is often caused by gastroesophageal reflux, where the stomach acid refluxes, or regurgitates, back into the lower section of the esophagus. The lining of the esophagus is not the same as the lining of the stomach and cannot stand the acid's irritation. It is now believed that the lower esophageal sphincter (LES)—a sphincter is a band of muscle tissue that opens and closes entrances to body cavities—loses its ability to stay closed against the pressure of the stomach's contents, especially when a person is lying down. Thus, the pain—sometimes described as pressure or cramping—occurs most often about an hour after a meal or during sleep. The condition is related to hiatal hernia, where, because of an ostensible defect in the diaphragm muscles, a portion of the stomach sometimes is pushed up into the chest area, causing similar discomfort. At times the pain is so severe that a heart attack is erroneously suspected. When 100 consecutive patients with severe chest pains were studied, 77 complained of pain that was identical to that of angina (loss of oxygen to the heart). Sixteen of the 77 were ultimately diagnosed as having an esophageal problem.

One way to help determine if gastroesophageal reflux could be the cause of chest pain is to perform the string test. A gelatin capsule, filled with a 55-inch nylon string that has a loop on its free end, is swallowed with a small amount of water—much as medicine is taken—after the looped end of the string is fastened to the cheek by adhesive tape. Usually, two string tests are performed—one upon awakening or after fasting for at least four hours and the second about an hour following a filling meal. After 10 to 15 minutes, the string is pulled back up (the capsule at the end is made to detach at the slightest tug and then dissolves), and the string is tested for its pH, or acidity. It can also reveal bleeding in the upper portion of the gastrointestinal tract—esophagus, stomach or duodenum (beginning of the small intestine)—by showing flecks of red blood on the string as it is withdrawn (Figure 36).

A point of interest: the string, when left in place for three to four hours, can also be used to help detect certain parasites that are difficult to find in feces (see Gastrointestinal System Tests, **Feces Observations**)—giardiasis in particular, probably the most common cause of episodic diarrhea. Many doctors also send the recovered string to a laboratory to be examined for cancer cells and other intestinal infections.

You can estimate where portions of the string were located by measuring the distance from the teeth to the xiphoid process (the lowest point of the sternum), which lies over the esophagus. That part of the string that went through the stomach into the small intestine is usually a greenish brown color

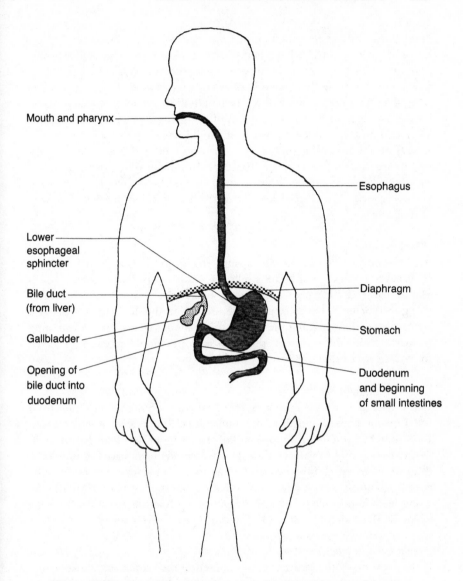

Figure 36. Bodily areas and locations involved with the string test.

after having been stained by bile. The portion of the string in between the two designated areas will have been in the stomach. For an average-sized adult, the first 15 inches of string from the teeth usually represent the esophagus; from 15 to 21 inches, the stomach; and the stained remainder, the duodenum (the first part of the small intestines).

What Is Usual

After the string has remained in the upper gastrointestinal tract for 15 minutes and has been retrieved, it is immediately stroked with a special pH (acidity-detecting) indicator stick and compared to its accompanying color chart. That portion of the string that rested in the esophagus should show a pH close to neutral, or a numerical value of 7. The length of string in the stomach should be acid—a value of 5 or less. The end of the string that passed through the stomach into the duodenum, where it should have been exposed to bile, is usually alkaline—a value of 7 or greater. If no food had been eaten for several hours prior to the test, the string should remain white (except for possible bile staining); eating within an hour before the test can cause flecks of partially digested food to stick to the string, but this does not interfere with acid testing.

What You Need

An Entero-Test, containing the capsule, string, pH indicator stick and pH color chart; a package of 25 tests sells for $72.00. A pediatric Entero-Test is also available at the same cost using a smaller-sized capsule and a shorter string (36 inches); this version can be used by adults for gastroesophageal reflux or blood testing, but the longer string should be used when searching for parasites in adults. A pocket light microscope, should you want to search for parasites, costs from $20.00 to $30.00.

What to Watch Out For

If you have had, or are having severe chest pain, do not attempt the string test until you have had medical attention and ruled out heart or lung disease. Be sure to tape the loose, looped end of the string to the cheek before swallowing the capsule. If you are going to leave the string in place for more than three hours to search for parasites, be sure to fast for at least four hours prior to testing and sip only water, if necessary, during the test period. Should the string seem impossible to retrieve, simply cut if off at the mouth and swallow it. No ill effects should occur, and you can repeat the test later.

What the Test Results Can Mean

If that portion of the string that was limited to the esophagus shows acidity (a pH of 6 or less), it could mean that stomach acid is escaping into the esophagus. Such a finding, especially if accompanied by heartburn–like symptoms, warrants a medical consultation. If the portion of the string in the stomach shows little or no evidence of any acid (a pH of 6 or greater), it could be a sign of pernicious anemia and also warrants a medical consultation. Thyroid disease, adrenal gland dysfunction and growths in the stomach can also cause a lack of acid in the stomach. Failure to see bile staining on that part of the string that should have gone through the stomach into the small intestines could indicate gallbladder or liver problems (see Urine Tests, **Bilirubin** test). Any sign of bleeding on the string, no matter where, warrants medical attention (see Gastrointestinal System Tests, **Feces Observations** for occult blood). If there is any doubt whether a pink or red stain on the string is blood, a Hemastix dipstick (see Urine Tests, **Blood** test) can be touched to the suspicious area. If parasites are suspected, a medical consultation should already have been sought. If the parasites have not been identified, rubbing that portion of the string that was in the small intestines on a glass slide and looking through a pocket light microscope could reveal a live parasite or its cyst (egg form). Identification of a parasite warrants medical attention.

GENITOURINARY SYSTEM TESTS

GONORRHEA

Gonorrhea is primarily an infection of the urethra (the passage that carries urine from the bladder to the outside of the body) (Figure 7); it is one of the most common sexually transmitted diseases (formerly called venereal diseases). Gonorrhea must be differentiated from non-gonococcal-caused urethritis; the latter is usually caused by a different microorganism called chlamydia. The treatment for the two similar symptom-causing conditions can be quite different, as are the potential consequences. Later complications of gonorrhea include urethral stricture, where the urethra must be surgically reopened, eye ulcers, throat infections, arthritis, heart disease, meningitis and, of course, sterility—especially in women. The most common symptoms are burning upon urination and a cream-to-yellow-colored discharge between one to three days after being infected; while men easily recognize the discharge at the end of the penis, most women are unaware that they have become infected until secondary damage begins. Although absolute diagnosis can only be obtained by growing the specific gonococcus germ in a culture, there are easy, quick, fairly reliable tests for men who have a penile discharge. A man has a one-in-four chance of contracting gonorrhea following one sexual act with an infected woman. A woman, on the other hand, has much more than a fifty-fifty chance of acquiring the disease after one sexual act with an infected man. This is because a man's infection is most often in the urethra and subsequent urination tends to eliminate the bacteria; a woman's infection is most often in the vagina where urination has no effect and where the bacteria tend to multiply and persist.

Incidentally, this disease is often referred to as "the clap," which comes from the colloquial use of a French word meaning house of prostitution. And not so incidentally, most states have laws that require any person (not just a physician) aware, or even suspicious, that he or she—or anyone else—has gonorrhea to report that fact to the public health authorities.

What Is Usual
There should be no evidence that gonorrhea could be present; in fact, there should be no urethral discharge.

What You Need
A watch and a Gonodecten test kit, which costs from $4.50 to $5.00, are required. This is considered a presumptive test, for it works on the principle of a color change within three minutes if a drop of urethral discharge contains gonorrheal bacteria; it is not absolutely specific for that germ, however, and on rare occasions could show a positive reaction with a similar, but nonvenereal, infection. Complete, easy-to-follow instructions are included with each test kit.

Another home-test gonorrhea kit is called VD Alert. While this test will soon be available in pharmacies, information can be obtained from the company, Medical Frontier Enterprises, P.O. Box 254, Bellbrook, Ohio, 45305. Here, a drop of urethral discharge is placed on a glass slide and mailed to the company with a private code number. After sufficient time for mail delivery and laboratory microscopic examination (usually two to three days), the sender of the slide calls a toll-free number and is told the result of the test: positive, negative, inconclusive (a nongonorrhea infection exists) or no result (improperly prepared or damaged slide), with the company offering a replacement kit without charge. At present the kit, with all necessary equipment and mailing container, costs $14.95. No personal identification is ever required.

What to Watch Out For
- The tests are for men only, at this time
- Do not urinate for at least one hour prior to performing the test
- If you have taken antibiotics prior to the test, they can cause a false-negative result
- Do not touch any part of the body with the test material
- Be extremely careful when obtaining a discharge specimen; it could be infected
- Do not engage in any form of sexual activity until you know you are free of disease.

What the Test Results Can Mean
A positive result with either test is considered at least 95 percent accurate in indicating gonorrhea; immediate medical attention is warranted. Because of the greatly increased chance of catching syphilis along with gonorrhea, a positive gonorrhea test should offer sufficient motivation to have a test for syphilis once a month for the next six months. But even a negative test for gonor-

rhea in the presence of a urethral discharge warrants medical attention to arrive at a specific diagnosis in order to prevent dangerous complications (see Urine Tests, **Leukocyte** and **Nitrite** tests); what are you waiting for?

MURPHY'S SIGN

Many people simply endure what seems to be a chronic backache—uncomfortable, but not sufficiently painful to seek medical consultation. In most instances, the cause is a muscle strain from overexertion or exercise. But a backache can also signal the beginning of kidney disease, most likely an infection around the outside of the kidney. The sooner a kidney problem is detected and treated, the less chance for permanent kidney damage and uremia—an extremely toxic condition that can require dialysis and even be fatal. Repeated testing for Murphy's sign whenever a backache occurs can be lifesaving.

The kidneys are located within the abdominal portion of the body toward the back and just under the ribs. To be more specific, they lie just under the skin of the back where the lowest (12th) rib joins the spinal column; the area is called the costovertebral angle (*costo* pertains to the ribs; *vertebral* refers to the spinal column). Some doctors refer to this area as the costophrenic angle, because it is also where the 12th rib lies adjacent to the diaphragm (*phrenic* refers to the diaphragm). Usually, the left kidney is a bit higher than the right, because of the liver's location just above the right kidney.

If the kidney is infected, it usually swells, and a mild blow over the costovertebral angle with the side of a closed fist will likely elicit a sensation of pain or severe discomfort (Figure 37).

What Is Usual
A moderate thump over the costovertebral angle (whether self-administered or performed by another) should elicit no discomfort at all.

What You Need
A few minutes are required to feel your back and locate the costovertebral angle; follow the bottom edge of the lowest rib until it joins the spine.

What to Watch Out For
Do not hit too hard; a forceful blow is not necessary when the kidney is infected. Of course, if you are very obese, it may be hard to pinpoint the costovertebral angle, but a blow to the general area should still elicit acute discomfort different from the dull ache of muscle strain.

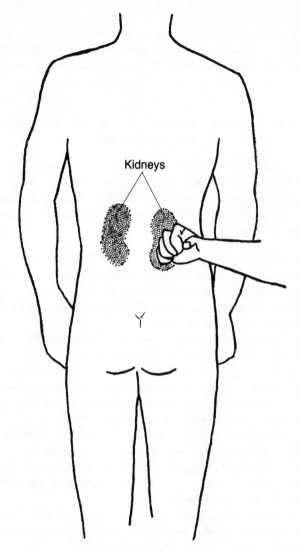

Figure 37. Murphy's sign.

What the Test Result Can Mean
A positive Murphy's sign (a sharp pain when the costovertebral angle is thumped) warrants medical attention. Most often this means a kidney infection, but it could also reflect other kidney pathology. (See Urine Tests, **Blood**, **Leukocyte** and **Nitrite** tests.) A colicky pain in the same area (intermittent

and not necessarily related to movement) without the need for thumping is one sign of kidney stones.

(*Note:* Some physicians use the term *Murphy's sign* for yet another physical examination test: They push their fingers under the right front ribs and have the patient take a deep breath; if this causes pain, it can mean gallbladder disease.)

NOCTURNAL PENILE TUMESCENCE SCREENING (STAMP TEST FOR IMPOTENCE)

Impotence means the inability to achieve an erection of the penis; it has nothing to do with fertility, or the ability to cause pregnancy. Although the condition was once thought to be almost always psychological, it has now been shown that a substantial number of men suffer impotence due to an organic or physical problem:

- Impotence may be secondary to a seemingly unrelated disease, such as diabetes, where subsequent atherosclerosis can interfere with the blood supply to the penis or where diabetes-caused impairment of nerve impulse transmission occurs; leukemia, Peyronie's disease and even sickle-cell anemia can also be to blame.
- An old, seemingly unrelated injury or previous surgery on the pelvis or spinal cord can be the underlying cause.
- The problem can be caused by testosterone deficiency, which can be the result of normal aging but can also come from pituitary disease; thyroid imbalance; adrenal conditions that interfere with, or even increase, cortisone production; or simply testicle dysfunction.
- Prostate problems—especially growths, but also as a consequence of some sexually transmitted disease—can also be responsible.
- Smoking and other lung problems have been shown to be associated with impotence (see Breath and Lung test; **Pulmonary Function Measurements; Breath Carbon Monoxide**)
- The repeated use of certain hair preparations, especially those that claim to grow hair may be an overlooked factor; some contain estrogens (female hormones)
- Drugs are probably the most common cause, with anything from large amounts of alcohol (colloquially referred to as "distiller's droop"), to normal doses of sedatives, tranquilizers, antianxiety and antidepressant medicines, small amounts of narcotics and just about any drug used to treat high blood pressure having been shown to prevent erection as a side effect. Some other medications also known to be a fault, although not as frequently, include: anticholinergics and other atropinelike drugs; antihistamines; estrogens (which may be part of certain meats if the ani-

mals were fattened by hormones); toxic-producing fungi (mycotoxins such as zearalenone) that can grow on improperly stored grains such as corn or wheat and if eaten, act as if they were estrogens or female hormones (some doctors feel the oil in certain vitamin E capsules could contain the toxin); some preparations used to treat cancer, glaucoma and parasites; a few antibiotics; Cimetidine (a form of antihistamine used to treat ulcers); and drugs to treat parkinsonism (incidentally, many of these drugs can also cause frigidity in women).

The basic test to help distinguish physical from psychological impotence is penile tumescence monitoring, usually performed in hospital sleep disorder centers, where measuring devices record the number and degree of penile erections that occur during sleep. It is considered normal for a man to have from one to four penile erections intermittently throughout the night when the deepest stage of sleep takes place—called REM sleep because it occurs along with *r*apid *e*ye *m*ovements, which take place at the same time. Such professional testing is quite expensive, and many doctors suggest that patients worried about impotence first perform the stamp test at home.

Just prior to retiring, a strip of several stamps connected only by perforations at each side is placed around the base of the flaccid penis so that the first is glued over the last to make a closed ring. The stamps are then examined the next morning, on awakening, to see if any of the perforations along the side were torn open—an indication that at least one erection probably took place during sleep (Figure 38). The test should be repeated for three nights.

What Is Usual
It is considered normal for the stamps to tear during the night (indicating an erection during sleep). Nocturnal erections normally tend to lessen after the age of 50 but should still occur occasionally.

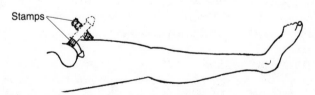

NPT	NPT	NPT	NPT	NPT	NPT	NPT	NPT	NPT	NPT

Strip of Nocturnal penile tumescence stamps as manufactured at the Oregon Health Sciences University

Stamps

Figure 38. Nocturnal penile tumescence screening.

What You Need

A strip of stamps or segments of glue-backed paper connected only by perforations at the side is required; while the post office sells a ready-made roll of one hundred 20-cent stamps for $20.00, you can make a similar, far-less-expensive device by asking a postal clerk to tear off one or more horizontal strips of 1-cent stamps from their standard sheets of 100. Mention must be made of a recent article in a medical journal that reports that postal officials require you to obtain permission from the Secret Service in the Treasury Department in order to use postage stamps for such testing. That same article also notes that use of Christmas Seals for this purpose requires permission from the American Lung Association. Some stationery stores carry glue-backed, or gummed, sheets of address labels that are separated by perforations. And as of now there seem to be no restrictions on the use of trading stamps.

The Oregon Health Sciences University Printing Service sells nocturnal penile tumescence (NPT) screening stamps; a minimum order of 10 sheets of 90 stamps at a cost of $1.00 per sheet is required. Checks should be made out to the Urology Gift Account, #70–262–2846; the cost is tax-deductible.

For those who simply cannot bring themselves to consider strips of stamps as professional scientific equipment, there is the Dacomed Snap-Gauge, a specially designed, padded, cloth and plastic band that is fastened around the penis with Velcro straps. This device not only reacts to an enlargement of the penis, it also contains three separately colored built-in snap elements that are set to break at different levels of rigidity, thus revealing a much more precise measure of intercourse capability which would be considered perfectly normal if all three snap elements break during the night. Although this device does not require a prescription, and can be performed in the privacy of one's home, it is advisable to obtain the Snap-Gauge through a physician or sex counselor. They cost $25.00 each and are made by the Dacomed Corporation, 1701 East 79th Street, Minneapolis, MN 55420. When compared to the usual $1,000.00 a night charge by impotence testing laboratories, the cost is relatively minor; some health insurance companies will reimburse you for the cost of the Snap-Gauge when used under a doctor's direction.

What to Watch Out For

Check that the perforations tear easily; some postage stamps today are difficult to tear apart. Do not use alcohol or take any sedatives or sleeping medicines for at least two days before testing; these drugs tend to prevent REM sleep, during which nocturnal erections are most apt to occur.

What the Test Results Can Mean

Tearing of the strip of stamps during the night usually means an erection took place. If erections are impossible at other times, the chances are the problem is psychological, and a medical consultation is warranted. Failure of the stamps to tear over a three-night period can mean there is some physical condition or drug interference causing impotence, and a medical consultation is warranted to help detect the underlying condition or to uncover the dastardly drug. If the Dacomed Snap-Gauge is used, the results are best interpreted by your physician.

PROSTATE OBSERVATIONS

The prostate, a small gland found only in men, is considered an integral part of the reproductive system because of its chemical and enzyme secretions, which increase during sexual activity. It is located just under the bladder at the point adjacent to where the urethra begins (the urethra is the tube that carries urine from the bladder through the penis to the outside). The prostate is also adjacent to the wall of the rectum, about three inches from the anus.

Normally the prostate stays the same size until around the age of 50, after which it almost always grows larger, so that by the age of 70 virtually every man has some degree of enlargement. Unfortunately, such enlargement sometimes makes urination difficult in various ways. It may be a strain to start urinating; the normal force of urination may be lessened; or it may seem that the amount of urine is diminished, causing a need to urinate more often. Such conditions can cause urine to remain in the bladder for longer periods than usual and can lead to bladder or kidney infection. (See Urine Tests, **Leukocyte** and **Nitrite** tests.) Although most men become consciously aware when the force of urination seems less than usual, there is an easy medical test that will show the peak urinary flow rate in numerical values, allowing a more precise evaluation of any urinary blockage that might be due to prostate enlargement (see Urine Tests, **Urine Flow Rate** test). An enlarged or infected prostate may also be the cause of blood in the urine (see Urine Tests, **Blood** test). Then there is the possibility of a cancer developing in the gland; it is estimated that 60,000 American men will have such a cancer diagnosed each year, and no one knows how many go undiagnosed. The earlier an enlarged or nodular prostate gland is detected and cause determined, the easier the treatment and the fewer the consequences.

While there are many sophisticated chemical blood and urine tests to help diagnose prostate disease, the digital rectal examination is still considered the most sensitive and efficient of all prostate tests. Many partners have learned to perform this simple examination semiannually to the satisfaction and inner security of all parties.

What You Need

The test requires a thin latex, rubber or plastic glove (disposable plastic gloves that fit any size hand are best; latex gloves cost $10.00 per 100, and disposables cost $5.00 per 100); some lubricant such as glycerine, plain (*not* carbo-lated) petroleum jelly or petrolatum (Vaseline is one brand name; K-Y Jelly, which doctors prefer, costs $1.00 a tube and is another similar product); and patience and understanding between examiner and examinee.

What Is Usual

After the person whose prostate is to be examined bends over a table or bed with the stomach and chest down on the surface (the knees may be bent to suit the level of table or bed), the examiner lubricates the gloved finger and gently presses it against the anus at first, without trying to insert it (Figure 39). Repeated light pressure will allow the finger to enter the rectum more easily than a sudden, forceful insertion attempt. Once the finger is inside the rectum to its full length, it is moved lightly back and forth over the anterior rectal surface (toward the abdominal side). The prostate gland should feel about 1 to 1¼ inches in size (some doctors describe it as walnut-sized), and it usually protrudes against the wall of the rectum. With a normal-sized pros-tate, a shallow vertical groove is commonly felt in the midline between the two lobes on either side that make up the smooth posterior surface of the

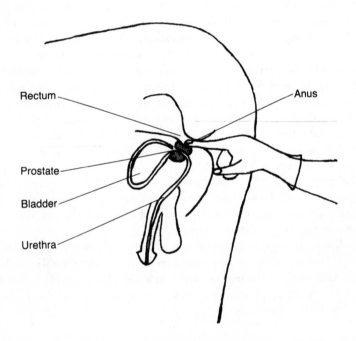

Figure 39. Prostate examination.

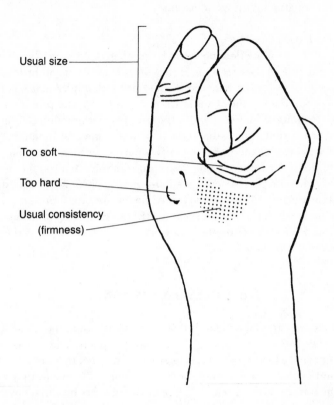

Usual size

Too soft

Too hard

Usual consistency
(firmness)

Figure 40. Making a fist to approximate the prostate gland's size and consistency.

gland. If you make a very tight fist and feel the soft but firm area between the base of the thumb and the base of the index finger, it approximates normal prostate consistency (Figure 40).

When the finger is lightly pressed from the outer margins of the prostate toward the center or midline portion repeatedly, it simulates a prostate massage, often employed when performing the urine **Two/Three-Glass** test.

What to Watch Out For
• The bladder and the bowels should be emptied prior to examination
• The examining finger should not have a long, sharp fingernail
• Do not use medicated ointment for a lubricant

• Do not force the entrance of the examining finger; if strong resistance is felt, do not attempt the examination.

What the Test Results Can Mean

If the size of the prostate does not seem larger than the distance between the tip of the thumb and the first joint, if the consistency is not soft or mushy, if the midline groove can be felt, and if there are no nodules that feel like a hard, bony thumb joint, the chances are reasonable that the prostate is as it should be. If, however, there is any suspicion of something different in size, shape, texture or smoothness, that is the time to seek medical attention. Many doctors will use this examination to verify a partner's observations and confirm the findings for future testing. Some doctors will use a routine medical checkup to teach the prostate examination—but usually only on request.

Note: Many doctors will touch the gloved finger used for a prostate examination to an occult blood test kit such as HEMATEST (see Gastrointestinal System Tests, **Feces Observations**) to perform an occult blood test at the same time. You can do the same.

TESTICLE OBSERVATIONS

The testicles are egg-shaped glands that lie in the scrotum, the skin-covered sac that hangs between a man's legs, just below the penis. The two testes are the male gonads, which produce sperm and testosterone; they correspond to the egg and estrogen-producing ovaries in a woman. Normally, they are in place at the time of birth, although in one or two of every hundred boys, they may not descend from the groin area for two or three weeks after birth. They generally do not become active until after 12 years of age. The testicles are subject to infections, varicose veins, hernias, edema, cysts and tumors. Regular examination of the scrotum and testicles is comparable to regular self-examination of the breasts in women; the earlier any seeming abnormality is discovered, the better the prognosis. While testicular cancer is the most common cancer of young men, it is also one of the few cancers that, when detected early, has a high cure rate with drugs.

First, stand in front of a mirror and observe the size and symmetry of each testicle in the scrotum. Then, with one foot resting on an elevated surface, apply the thumb and fingertips to the scrotal sac opposite the raised leg (Figure 41). Gently roll each testicle between the thumb and fingers until all surfaces have been inspected. Next, in a darkened room, place the tip of a flashlight behind, and in the center of, each testicle and note the amount and dispersion of the light shining around the testicle through the scrotal sac (Figure 42).

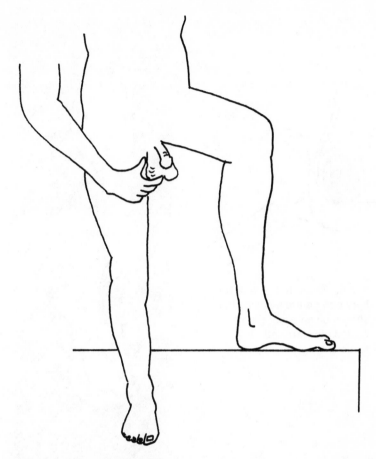

Figure 41. Testicle examination (when examining a testicle, it is best to raise the opposite foot off the floor).

What Is Usual

When standing in front of a mirror, both testicles in the scrotum should appear egg-shaped and the same size, although it is common for the left testicle to be slightly lower than the right. The evident surface of each testicle should appear smooth, with no bumps, nodules or bulges showing. When palpated (examined by touch), each testicle should be about two inches long, very smooth on the surface, with a firm, spongelike consistency. Above the testicle a cordlike structure (the spermatic cord, containing the epididymus and vas deferens, which carry sperm to the penis) is felt going into the groin area. It is not unusual for the testicle and cord to be quite sensitive to palpation, especially

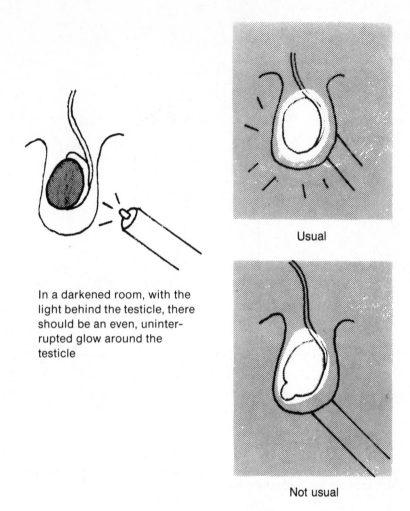

Usual

In a darkened room, with the
light behind the testicle, there
should be an even, uninterrupted glow around the
testicle

Not usual

Figure 42. Testicle transillumination.

when this examination is performed for the first time. With a bright light behind the scrotum and each testicle, the testicle itself appears as a smooth, oval, dark shadow surrounded by an even, red glow. As the light is moved about the scrotum, no other shadows or irregularity in the testicle's shape should be seen.

What You Need
The test requires a penlight type of flashlight with a small bulb or small, bright light source; an area that can be darkened; and a low stool (or a few

books) upon which to rest one foot. The twin transilluminator, described in the **Sinus Transillumination** test, will also work well for this test.

What to Watch Out For
Do not try to examine your testicles if you are in a cold environment; cold temperatures cause the scrotum to shrink in size and can hinder a proper examination. Do not be too delicate when palpating, or small nodules might be overlooked; but if the spermatic cord seems unusually tender, it could indicate the beginning of an infection called epididymitis, and immediate medical attention is warranted. Do not attempt a testicle examination if you have been exposed to someone with mumps or think you might have the disease.

What the Test Results Can Mean
If, after your first testicle examination, you can have your own observations confirmed by your doctor, and the results indicate normal testicles, you can achieve great peace of mind by performing this test monthly and uncovering no possible abnormalities. Should one scrotal side appear larger and somewhat pear-shaped, but still allow the transmission of light, it could be the start of a hydrocele, or excessive fluid surrounding the testicle, a slow-developing condition that warrants a medical consultation. A somewhat similar condition that feels like worms around the testicle and usually does not allow light transmission could be the beginning of varicose veins from the spermatic cord; it, too, warrants a medical consultation. If either or both testicles feel smaller than 1½ inches long, this could reflect an inherited condition but may also reflect a hormone dysfunction. Should you have edema (water retention) elsewhere in your body, such as around your ankles, it is not uncommon for the scrotal sacs to swell up with fluid as well. But most of all, you should be on the lookout for any hard, especially painless, node or bump that interferes with the usual smooth surface of the testicle, and particularly a lump—no matter how tiny—that does not allow light transmission. Such a test result warrants immediate medical attention.

If you know you had one or both testicles undescended at birth, even if they later descended by themselves or were surgically repaired, you should be aware of the statistics that indicate you have a 40 times greater chance of developing testicular cancer than men born with descended testicles. Men with such a medical history should be even more careful to perform testicle observations monthly starting at 15 years of age.

MISCELLANEOUS TESTS

ALLERGY PATCH TESTING AND ELIMINATION DIET

Patch testing to detect allergic or hypersensitivity reactions was first tried nearly 100 years ago; it is still considered a valuable, if not precise, evaluation of an individual's immune system response to provocation. When an antigen (bacteria, virus, parasite, poison, pollen, chemical or unfamiliar protein such as may be found in food) enters the body, it can provoke the production of specific antibodies by certain body organs. These antibodies, now known to be immunoglobulins, circulate through the blood to where the antigens have settled; in the case of allergy, it may be in the lungs, causing asthma; in the skin, causing a rash; in the bowels, causing diarrhea; or in the nose, causing sneezing and mucus production—to name but a very few manifestations. If one's immunity is in good working order, the antibodies help prevent disease or allergic symptoms.

The patch test is a means of applying a suspected allergy-causing antigen to the skin's surface to see if it provokes an antibody response. Although this test really only measures the response of the skin, some doctors feel it can offer valuable clues to other allergic-type bodily responses—asthma, bloodshot eyes, eczema, hay fever, headaches, hyperactivity, runny nose, sinusitis, stomach cramps, diarrhea, urticaria (hives) and even personality changes such as learning difficulties and bizarre behavior.

The patch test is almost identical to the intradermal skin test, the exception being that no needle injection is made just under the surface of the skin. Instead, a very small amount of the potentially allergenic substance (about the size of the head of a match) is placed on a half-inch circle or square of gauze; if it is not already in liquid form, mix it well into one or two drops of water or mineral oil—the oil will not evaporate, as water sometimes does. The wet patch of gauze is then placed against the skin and covered with adhesive tape; unmedicated Band-Aid-type adhesive bandages have the gauze patch built in and work well. Use skin surfaces where there is no hair, such as the inside of the arm or the back. Leave the patch in place for two days (48 hours), and try not to let it become wet. If, however, the skin under the patch starts to itch, burn, ache or feel irritated in any way, no matter how slight, remove the patch immediately and wash the area well with water. Should the irritation continue, apply a nonprescription cortisone ointment and consult your physician.

After the patch is removed, your susceptibility to the substance applied is supposedly indicated by how much redness, swelling, papules (pimples), vesicles (blisters) and itching are present (Figure 43) on the skin where it was in

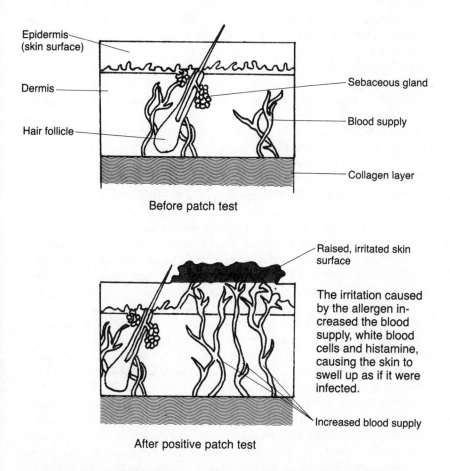

Epidermis
(skin surface)

Dermis

Hair follicle

Sebaceous gland

Blood supply

Collagen layer

Before patch test

Raised, irritated skin surface

The irritation caused by the allergen increased the blood supply, white blood cells and histamine, causing the skin to swell up as if it were infected.

Increased blood supply

After positive patch test

Figure 43. Allergy Patch Testing—diagrammatic cross-section view of the skin before patch test is applied and after positive patch test. The skin consists of two distinct layers, with the epidermis being the surface layer. Under the dermis layer is subcutaneous tissue, which includes collagen (the protein fibers that act as a matrix to hold tissues and organs together).

contact with the antigen (see Miscellaneous Tests, **Skin Observations**). A skin response (positive reaction, in which the surface of the skin is raised and usually red where it came into contact with the allergy-provoking substance) may not appear for anywhere from one hour to two additional days after the patch is removed, so the skin test site should be examined for up to two days afterward. If no signs of irritation are seen, it is then considered a negative reaction (Figure 43). It has been observed that positive immediate reactions (irritation before the patch was supposed to be removed) are more apt to come from allergies to drugs or foods, while allergies to plants, pollens and pets seem to take longer to show themselves. Positive delayed reactions are also thought to be indicative of a poorly functioning immune system and may suggest an increased susceptibility to disease in general.

Should you attempt patch testing for the first time, always place two additional identical patches, one patch completely dry and another soaked with the water or oil used to mix with the test substance—but both without the test substance—on different areas of the skin to be sure you are not allergic to the gauze, adhesive tape or diluting liquid. If either of the "control" patches shows a positive reaction, the allergy test cannot be considered accurate, and different materials should be tried.

It is quite possible to test for several different allergy-provoking substances at the same time, but each patch should be kept well separated from the others. If a negative response appears in the face of a very suspicious substance, it may be that the amount of test substance was insufficient to provoke a reaction; try the test again a week later with twice as much material.

When selecting test material for allergy patch testing, start out with the most common allergy-causing substances. With foods, milk, eggs (most often only the white part) and wheat flour are frequently to blame. Should bread provoke a positive reaction, you may have to retest using the specific grains from which the flour was made; then again, an allergy can come from other added ingredients. In some cases, it turns out not to be the food that causes the allergy but rather the chemicals that restaurants and food processors use on and in foods to keep them looking fresh, enhance flavor, provide color and prevent spoilage (e.g., sulfites; tartrazine, or FD&C yellow No. 5—a food coloring; monosodium glutamate).

Testing for an allergy to pets requires a bit of animal hair or feathers; sometimes a drop or two of saliva will provoke a more specific reaction. Birds seem to cause far more allergies than is generally suspected, and they spread their symptom-producing substances throughout a room every time they preen themselves and flap their wings—even while in their cages.

Pollen testing may be difficult when grasses, trees and weeds are involved, for you should try to isolate the specific pollen; if this is not possible, you can use a bit of grass or leaves, but be sure they have not been sprayed with pesticides, fertilizers or other chemicals. Obtaining pollen from house plants and flowers should be less of a problem.

While drugs are the most common cause of allergic reactions, drug allergies are also the easiest to test for. You must use extreme caution, however, when evaluating sensitivity to medicines, for sometimes the tiniest trace of a drug—especially a penicillin product—can cause a severe reaction. In addition animal feed can contain several drugs, especially antibiotics, and at times animals are dipped in antibiotic solutions after slaughter; eating meat from such animals can also provoke an allergic reaction. Never test yourself for a drug allergy if you know you are already allergic to any other drug.

Other common allergy-provoking substances include: house dust, cotton linters and other upholstery and mattress-stuffing materials—even the stuffing in toys, various fabrics, tobacco smoke, insecticides, paints, cosmetics, deodorants, toothpaste, detergents, molds and smog; the list is virtually endless.

The purpose of patch testing is not only to detect allergy-provoking substances but, more important, to enable you to eliminate them from your lifestyle if at all possible. This, of course, is not always easy; if the family pet turns out to be the guilty party, simply putting that pet in another home might not result in any improvements until all traces of the animal's hair and saliva and everything that the hair or saliva came in contact with is also removed. It is usually easier to change the environment of the allergic person to one where no pets are kept and see what happens in a week or so. If a specific household product turns out to be the cause of an allergy, removal of the substance might be rewarded by symptom relief within days. With pollen-type allergies, desensitization may be attempted, but it is not always successful; avoidance of the pollen through electronic filtered air conditioning may help, but usually total removal of the pollen source, or removal of the person from the pollen source, is the only successful treatment.

Elimination diet. When it comes to food allergies, the logical next step after a positive patch test for a specific food is to eliminate the suspect food or foods from the diet and see if annoying or irritating symptoms disappear. Elimination diet testing can be performed without previous patch testing, especially if there are strong suspicions about one or more foods. A successful elimination diet test not only requires elimination of the suspect food for several weeks but seems to work best if, during the first few days, only commonly known foods that rarely provoke allergy are eaten: rice, tea (only beet sugar should be used; cane sugar is a known allergen). A careful, written record should be kept of all foods eaten. After four to seven days, one suspect food is introduced back into the diet every two days, and symptomatic allergic reactions, if they occur, are noted. The most common symptoms provoked by this test particularly include: indigestion, stomach cramps, heartburn, headache, hyperactivity, runny nose, skin rash, unusual behavior and even edema (water retention, causing puffiness of the face, hands or feet). In the face of an allergy within 1 to 10 hours after eating a suspect food, omit that food again for four days and then try it once more; another allergic response justifies elimination of that food from the diet. Of course, the degree of symptom aggravation must be weighed against the degree of pleasure derived from the food, and only the allergic individual can make such a decision. When milk products are reintroduced into the diet, a distinction must be made between milk allergy and milk intolerance (see Gastrointestinal System Tests, **Milk Products [Lactose] Intolerance** test).

Some other simple tests that can hint at an underlying allergy include:

* The Tang test—after drinking a six-ounce glass of Tang (or any other products whose label lists the coloring "FD&C yellow No. 5," which is really tartrazine), hypersensitive individuals will usually show an allergic reaction such as asthma; tartrazine is contained in hundreds of food products: commercial desserts, cake mixes, candies, seasonings, packaged dinners, ice creams and sherbets, salad dressings, the coatings around medicines and vitamin pills, etc.
* Dermatographism—stroking the skin, usually on the back, with a dull instrument may produce weltlike urticarial lesions (raised white plaques or flat patches surrounded by red areas) where the instrument stroked
* Cold response—ice placed against the skin may produce an urticarial rash similar to dermatographism
* Sunlight response—sunlight may cause a dermatographism-type rash. When people are suspected of having an allergic reaction to sunlight, they are usually asked to expose themselves to bright sunlight through a window glass to see if the window blocks out the sun's allergy-causing rays
* Stress response—people who develop a dermatographism-type rash when they are upset or subject to anxiety usually develop a similar allergic rash after strenuous physicial activity; a stress-type allergy can sometimes be confirmed by having the patient exercise vigorously and then noting the appearance of a rash immediately afterward
* Pressure response—a dermatographism-type rash may develop on the arms after heavy bundles have been carried; a similar rash may develop on the buttocks after a person has been sitting for several hours
* Water response—a dermatographism-type rash may occur over the upper part of the body within 15 minutes after a warm bath.

Allergic reactions must sometimes be differentiated from other types of skin reactions such as herpes (see Miscellaneous Tests, **Skin Observations**), parasite infestations (see Miscellaneous Tests, **Skin Infestation—Flea Bites**, **Skin Infestation—Pediculosis** and **Skin Infestation—Scabies**), eczema, generalized itching from sweat or high humidity (prickly heat), and manifestations of some systemic disease (liver disease; certain cancers; kidney disease; thyroid disease; and polycythemia, a disease involving the production of too many red blood cells).

What Is Usual
Any allergy is not really normal; unfortunately, many people inherit their allergic tendency, and while not normal, it is still "usual" for such an individual.

What You Need
The test requires small, square or round gauze pads (cotton-filled Quick-Pads will also work); adhesive tape (if you already know you are allergic to adhesive tape, you might try Dermicel, Trico-Mesh or some other hypo-allergenic tape). Band-Aid and Telfa brands of spots or square bandages are preferable because they have adhesive tape all around the gauze, but strip Band-Aid types will still work. Small Coverlet brand adhesive dressings work very well. A tube of a cortisone skin cream or ointment may also be needed should skin irritation occur.

What to Watch Out For
You should be alert for any intense allergic response; do not leave any patch test on if any irritation, no matter how slight, occurs. Use a patch that will not allow easy evaporation of the liquid—that is, one that is not too porous. If at all possible, try to keep the test substance free of any contamination. Never leave a patch test on for more than 48 hours, but be sure to continue watching the test area for at least two days after removing the patch. If you know you are already allergic, or seem to have allergy-type reactions to many substances, check with your doctor before attempting any patch test. Do not attempt patch testing if you have any skin irritation, such as a sunburn or skin infection. Do not rub or put any pressure on the patch while it is in place or on the test area after the patch has been removed; it can cause a false-positive reaction. If you are taking any antiallergy medicine, such as antihistamines or cortisone products, check with your doctor before testing; they can cause false-negative reactions.

Keep in mind that certain areas of your body may be more sensitive than others; many people find the back twice as sensitive as the inner part of the upper arm. Some people find that when they apply patch tests early in the morning, they seem to have a greater, more immediate response than when they are applied in the afternoon. And if the patches are too near each other, a positive test with one patch can cause a false-positive test in an adjacent patch.

What the Test Results Can Mean
A positive patch test usually, but not always, indicates something to which you are allergic. When subsequent avoidance or elimination of that substance brings relief from allergy symptoms, the test has been successful. The same principle applies to the elimination diet. Again, a positive skin-patch test may reflect only the skin's allergic response; it may not always be of value for pinpointing

the cause of other allergic symptoms. And a negative patch test does not always rule out an allergy. Evidence of allergy that cannot be controlled by avoidance or elimination warrants a medical consultation. Positive allergic patch test responses within minutes, or even within an hour, warrant medical attention; you could be so unusually sensitive that you require an antiallergy kit on hand at all times, together with the knowledge of how to use it. Doctors now have radioimmunosorbent assay (RAST) tests, which can help confirm an allergy, especially food reactions. Other indications of allergy such as dermatographism or a seemingly allergic response to water warrant a medical consultation to search for some possible underlying disease; itching after a bath is a common symptom of polycythemia (too many red blood cells).

Many people who are allergic to tartrazine are also allergic to aspirin and aspirin-containing medicines. Conversely, those with a known allergy to aspirin are frequently allergic to tartrazine.

Should you ultimately prove to suffer from an allergy, be sure to carry with you, or wear, some sort of identification to notify others of that fact. This is particularly important if you are allergic to a drug such as penicillin, and it can also help you avoid other problems related to hypersensitivity. (Contact the Medic–Alert Foundation, Turlock, CA. 95380.)

APNEA MONITORING

Apnea means the sudden involuntary stopping of breathing; it can last for a few seconds or for several minutes and it can be fatal. At this time there is no mutually agreed-upon reason for the condition, but the blame has been ascribed to:

- An obstruction somewhere in the bronchi, windpipe (trachea) or back of the throat; blockage of the breathing passage can come from enlarged tonsils, the tongue folding back on itself or a loss of tone in the throat muscles
- Hypersomnolence, or excessive sleeping, associated with the Pickwickian syndrome
- An upper respiratory infection (cold or flu), even a very slight one
- Heart rhythm irregularities
- Pathology in the part of the brain that controls respiration (resembling epilepsy, only without convulsions)
- Prematurity or low birth weight, especially if accompanied by anemia
- Hypoglycemia (see Blood Tests, **Glucose** test)
- Gastroesophageal reflux (see Gastrointestinal System Tests, **String Test**)
- Hormone-caused metabolic disorders
- Severe allergic reactions to almost everything, with dust and milk leading the list

• Smoking on the mother's part during pregnancy.

One form of the condition is called obstructive sleep apnea and is reportedly the most common cause of breathing failure during sleep. It consists of a periodic lack of breathing and interrupted sleeping and is believed to afflict more than 1 million Americans, 9 out of 10 of whom are men, most of them overweight, middle-aged and usually with high blood pressure (see Heart and Circulation Tests, **Blood Pressure** test), although a few young children with enlarged tonsils have had the problem.

The most common warning sign of sleep apnea in an adult is snoring—usually quite loud and of a sudden onset following quiet sleep; the snoring reflects the difficulty in breathing. While on occasion a bed partner's description of the snoring pattern can be an early warning sign of sleep apnea, some doctors advice patients suspected to have the condition to place a tape recorder next to the bed and record the snoring sounds during the night. After you later note the segments of the tape containing the snoring, your doctor can listen to those segments and, at times, make the diagnosis. More often than not, however, adult apnea is diagnosed in a hospital-based sleep disorder center where breathing and heart rate are recorded during snoring episodes.

A second form of sleep apnea occurs in infants, and from one to two out of every 1,000 babies—most commonly between two and four months of age—seem to suffer from this as yet indistinct condition. Some doctors consider sleep apnea to be the cause of the sudden infant death syndrome (SIDS), in which an infant who seemed in perfect health at night is found dead in bed the next morning (called cot death in England), but there is no professional pediatric consensus on this theory either. All that is agreed upon at this time is that any apnea in an infant lasting more than 20 seconds (or even less if there is any change in the infant's color from pink to paleness or blue, or if the heartbeat slows down) warrants immediate medical attention.

One phase of testing for sleep apnea, after initial medical studies indicate its possibility, is monitoring an infant's breathing and/or heart rate in the home 24 hours a day—especially while the infant is sleeping. Costwise, it is virtually prohibitive to perform the same task for several months in a hospital, where even specially trained nurses on eight-hour shifts in an intensive care setting using direct observation in place of monitors miss nearly 40 percent of apnea episodes. Battery-operated electronic detectors in pads are placed under the baby (in essence, they become the crib's mattress, although some do go beneath the mattress) or around the baby's chest as a nightshirt that constantly monitors every breath and/or heartbeat, no matter how slight. They do not require the attachment of wires or electrodes and do not actually touch the baby's skin. Respiration and heart rate are displayed on a connecting instrument as flashing lights, digital displays or through dial gauges. Your doctor can advise you which type would be best for your particular circumstances. The monitors detect any cessation of breathing or change in the heart rate and give off a loud alarm along with very bright flashing lights should breathing stop or the heart slow for 10 seconds (some monitors can be set to show apnea for anywhere from 5 to 20 seconds, depending on the doctor's recommendations; some have remote receivers that can be carried everywhere).

These monitors require special training, usually by the pediatrician or nurses in a hospital. It is necessary for parents to learn how to use the monitor and what to do should the alarm go off, as well as to receive counseling on the monitor's psychological impact on the whole family.

What Is Usual
Obviously, it is normal not to have any breathing difficulties. In this circumstance, however, the most common warning is a mother's seeing her child suddenly lose its usual skin color, at times even turn blue, and become limp and unresponsive.

What You Need
With the advice and cooperation of your physician, you can purchase or rent an infant sleep apnea monitor. There are many different kinds; some keep track of breathing only, while others also disclose the slightest change in the heartbeat. In general, the machines sell for $700.00 to $1600.00; they rent for $85.00 to $200.00 a month (in most instances they are not needed for more than two to three months). They are usually sold or rented through medical supply stores, such as Abbey Medical, although some hospitals also offer this service. Battery-powered machines are not subject to power failure. A tape recorder that records for several hours or someone to change the tape during the night.

What to Watch Out For
Most of all, you will have to deal with the potential tension that can come from having an infant sleep apnea monitoring machine in your home. Even though such stressful feelings cannot compare with the anxiety for the baby's condition, the machine's possible interference with family and social life can be emotionally traumatic. Be sure you know you will have adequate support from all family members at home; be equally sure all family members understand everything that home monitoring entails. Accept the fact that there will be false alarms; no machine is perfect. Do not become so dependent on the machine that you refuse to give it up when your doctor says it is no longer needed.

What the Test Results Can Mean
Ten years ago there were approximately 10,000 unexpected, sudden infant deaths believed to be related to sleep apnea each year. Where sleep apnea monitoring devices were properly used at home on children suspected of having the condition, the survival rate was almost 100 percent.

Any suspicion of sleep apnea in a child or adult (sudden episodes of loud snoring are considered an early warning sign) warrants medical attention; obstructive sleep apnea is a dangerous condition.

BODY TEMPERATURE

Body temperature is a manifestation of the body's metabolism; in actuality it reflects the heat produced by all sorts of body activities: digestion, breathing, hormone production, muscle activity (voluntary muscle movement such as when you move your arms and legs and involuntary muscle activity such as your heart beating) and even the formation of brain chemicals while thinking. When certain body activities (physical exercise, conversion of an excessive amount of food in the intestines, even fear) tend to raise your body temperature, you might start to perspire, and as your sweat evaporates, it acts as a cooling mechanism to counteract the temperature rise. In a cold environment, especially without adequate protection such as warm clothing, your muscles may start to tremble, and the shivering will help to raise your body temperature. Body temperature can be considered an indication of how efficiently your body is performing—much as with any other engine or machine. Although most people think almost exclusively of normal and elevated body temperature (fever), a lower-than-normal body temperature (hypothermia) can also point to certain diseases and even be life–threatening. Most often, however, a normal body temperature does signify good health, albeit there are exceptions (Figure 44).

A common cause of fever, not directly resulting from disease and frequently overlooked, comes from the use of certain drugs. Medicine taken for one purpose can have a secondary action, or side effect, of raising body temperature. Drug fever can be an early warning sign of an impending dangerous drug reaction and warrants immediate medical attention. A few examples of such drugs include: antibiotics, especially penicillin products and related drugs, sulfanilamide derivatives, streptomycin; antihistamines; procainamide, nicotinic acid and other vitamin B_3 derivatives; anticoagulants; iodine and iron compounds; barbiturates; most narcotics, especially cocaine; amphetamine products; a few drugs used to control heart rhythms; anticholinergic medications, including atropine; even aspirin products or several cups of caffeine-containing coffee, tea or cola drinks can indirectly raise body temperature. Your doctor or pharmacist can tell you if your medicines have this effect.

Ovulation time and fertility tests. In women the ovulation time test is performed by taking the body temperature daily on awakening (Figure 45). A small but significant rise in temperature (of one degree) midway between menstrual periods usually signals the time of ovulation (when an egg is expelled from an ovary to begin its journey to the uterus and when pregnancy

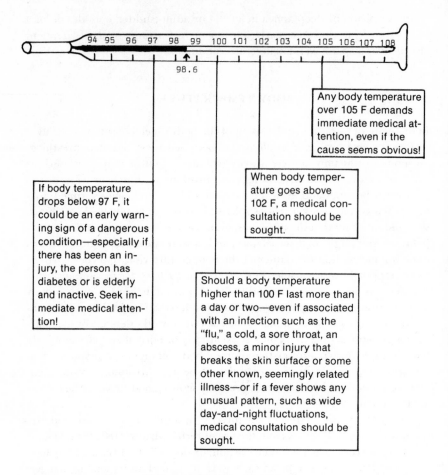

Figure 44. Body temperature.

is most likely to occur). The ovulation time test can also be used as a means of determining fertility; failure to show a rise in temperature between menstrual periods in a woman of childbearing age could indicate an inability to ovulate. Obviously, ovulation time can even be employed as a not-too-precise contraception technique by identifying those days when pregnancy should be impossible. Sometimes ovulation time measurements are called basal body temperature tests.

Spinnbarkeit test. Another confirmatory test for ovulation time is called *spinnbarkeit* (the word means threadiness), in which the viscosity (thickness or thinness) of mucus secreted by the cervix is observed. Remove some mucus from the vagina with your finger and place it between your thumb and first finger. Then, slowly spread the thumb and finger apart. Most of the time

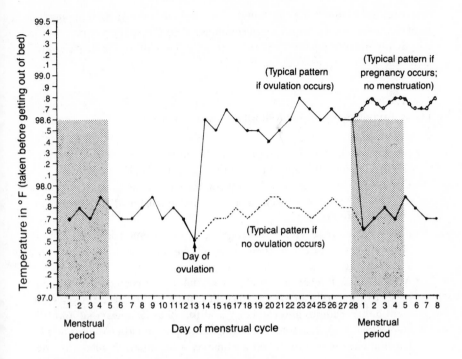

Figure 45. Typical ovulation time (basal body temperature) test pattern.

Note: During childbearing years the usual body temperature of a nonpregnant woman ranges between 97.5 F and 98 F.

during the menstrual cycle, the mucus is thick and sticky and will not stretch for more than an inch across the spreading fingers before breaking. A day before ovulation, and for a day or two afterward, however, when you are most able to become pregnant, the mucus becomes thin and watery and will easily stretch and remain as a long string between widely separated fingers. Some doctors consider this test more accurate than ovulation time-temperature measurements.

What Is Usual
Although the figure 98.6 F (37 C) is most often quoted as normal, most doctors take little notice of a body temperature ranging between 98 F (36.7 C) and 99.5 F (37.5 C) when the temperature is measured orally (with the thermometer under the tongue and the mouth closed). A rectally measured tem-

perature may be normal even though it is one-half to one degree higher. An axillary measurement (with the thermometer held under the armpit and the arm firmly pressed against the side) is usually one-half to one degree lower than oral temperatures when normal.

What You Need
The test requires one of the following types of thermometers:

- Glass and filled with mercury (usually silver-colored) or some other chemical (generally red); they cost from $1.00 to $4.00
- Electronic with a sensitive metal tip connected to a measuring device that displays the temperature on a scale or in digital form; they cost from $20.00 to $40.00
- A treated piece of paper with imprinted measurements, which is used once and then discarded; they come in boxes of 25 and cost from 10 to 25 cents each
- A STAT-TEMP fever detector; a small, flat, plastic coated circle that adheres to the forehead skin surface (it can be left in place for days for continuous readings and can be reused for 10 to 12 times) that immediately shows body temperature by digital display in either Centigrade or Fahrenheit; the manufacturer also makes a hypothermia model for detecting lower than normal body temperature; this can be very valuable for monitoring the elderly; they cost $1.95 each
- Special glass thermometers that read body temperature as low as 75° F (23.8° C) are available for $10.50 from Dynamed Inc., 6200 Yarrow Dr., Carlsbad, CA. 92008.

A special, easy-to-read ovulation thermometer costs approximately $4.00 and usually includes a pad of graph paper for recording daily readings. For those who do not want to bother with the work of measuring and recording ovulation time temperatures, a tiny computerized fertilization-time thermometer is available for approximately $40.00; after body temperature is taken, the device shows a green light when pregnancy is least likely.

Rectal temperature measurements are considered to be the most accurate (the thermometer should be left in place at least three minutes) but are really only necessary for infants or others who cannot hold a thermometer in the mouth; oral temperature measurements are sufficiently accurate for virtually all purposes; axillary and skin temperature measurements are the least accurate. Direct-reading thermometers, such as those with digital displays, while easier to read, are no more accurate than ordinary glass thermometers.

If a thermometer is not available, it is still possible to tell if someone has an elevated temperature by placing your palm or the back of your hand on your own forehead—assuming your body temperature is normal—and then comparing that with the degree of warmth felt on the forehead of the patient.

What to Watch Out For

Always make sure the thermometer reading is below normal before measuring body temperature. With the ordinary glass thermometer, lower the temperature reading to 95 F (35 C) by shaking the thermometer while holding the end opposite the measuring tip or bulb; or you can immerse the tip in cold water for a few minutes.

If you are particularly testing for hypothermia, be sure your thermometer will indicate readings as low as 94° F. (34.5° C.). A typical thermometer that must be shaken down before use has to have its indicator below 94° F before use; they usually do not drop below the temperature set by shaking down. If, after using such a thermometer, it shows no rise above 94° F immediate medical attention is warranted. For regular monitoring for hypothermia, a special low-reading thermometer, such as the STAT-TEMP mentioned above, should be used.

Unless the thermometer's accompanying instructions indicate otherwise, it should be left under the tongue or in the rectum for at least three minutes; if axillary measurements are made, the thermometer should remain well inside the armpit for at least five minutes.

When oral temperature is measured, do not eat, drink or smoke for at least one-half hour before testing and keep the mouth tightly closed for the entire time the thermometer is in place. Ideally, there should have been no physical activity for at least one hour prior to testing, no matter what technique is employed.

When recording ovulation time temperatures, they must be measured the first thing on awakening each morning before you get out of bed.

When you record the temperature, it is a good confirmatory measure to record the pulse rate (see Heart and Circulation Tests, **Pulse Measurements**) and the rate of breathing (respiration). Normally, the pulse rate and rate of breathing increase as body temperature rises.

Keep in mind that body temperature tends to be lower in the morning and higher toward evening.

If a body temperature reading does not seem to correspond with the patient's body warmth and other symptoms that usually accompany fever (flushed face, rapid pulse and breathing, lethargy), first check out the thermometer by measuring your own temperature or by comparing the reading with that of another thermometer. Should there still be some doubt, most doctors and hospitals verify their observations by measuring the temperature of a freshly passed urine sample.

What the Test Results Can Mean

If you know, or have good reason to suspect, that an infection exists, evidence of elevated body temperature (fever) is to be expected. Fever greater than 100° F (37.8C) warrants medical consultation. In most instances the degree of fever corresponds to the severity of the illness. As treatment is applied, the reduction of body temperature is a reasonable indication of the treatment's efficacy. On the other hand, if, after use of a prescribed antibiotic for more than 24 hours, there is no lowering of body temperature, this could be a warning that the drug is not effective, and immediate medical attention should be sought.

Should there be evidence of fever without any obvious or reasonable explanation (a recent fall or other injury, exposure to one of the many childhood illnesses or the residual effects of a return from foreign travel—some tropical-type diseases do not reveal themselves until weeks or months after exposure), then that fever could well be a first warning sign of a hidden kidney problem, a complication of liver metabolism or any of a hundred different conditions that warrant medical consultation.

At times fever reflects itself as night sweats—in which one wakes up during the night hot and sweat-soaked. Body temperature measurements may be close to normal during the day. Repeated bouts of night sweats usually come from low-grade infections, but they can also be a cancer warning sign; they warrant a medical consultation.

If a woman develops a fever during the first four weeks of pregnancy, she should immediately notify her doctor; it seems that a high fever in a pregnant woman can cause fetal development defects.

The pattern of fever during the day and over a period of several days may offer an important clue to a doctor as to the cause of an illness (Figure 46). The body temperature usually stays below 103 F (39.4 C) when a severe cold or pneumonia is caused by a virus; when the source of the infection is a bacteria or fungus, the fever is almost always higher than 103 F. When the fever seems close to normal every morning and then rises to more than 101 F (38.3 C) each evening, it could suggest brucellosis (sometimes called undulant fever), which can come from drinking raw milk. If a fever pattern stays high for several weeks without any usual dips, it can suggest psittacosis, a pneumonialike disease that can be caught from infected birds such as pigeons, parrots or parakeets. A fever chart that shows a very high temperature for a day or so, then a sudden drop for 12 to 24 hours, followed by another sharp rise, could make your doctor consider a hidden abscess. Malaria can show a high fever for anywhere from two to three days and then return to normal for a few days—depending on which of the four types of malaria a patient has contracted. Since many diseases have distinct fever patterns—especially when fever can be correlated with the pulse and respiration rates—it can be of great value to record these observations for your doctor.

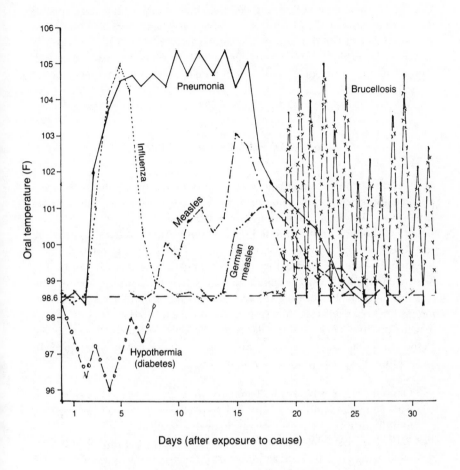

Figure 46. Some examples of disease fever patterns.

Because it is common for people over the age of 60 to have a normal temperature as low as 97.6° F (36.4 C), it is easy to miss accidental hypothermia (abnormally low body temperature)—from 95 F to 97° F (35 C to 36.1 C)—which can be extremely dangerous. As we become older, our body metabolism tends to slow down normally, and this, in turn, helps lower body temperature. Hypothermia as an illness may occur following an injury, along with malnutrition or dehydration, as an insulin reaction in patients with diabetes and even as a consequence of alcohol use. It is considered good preventive medicine to measure the body temperature of any elderly person daily—especially one who is living alone. People usually shiver and cannot perform some normal tasks when body temperature drops below 96 F (35.5 C). Below

95 F (35 C), there may be slurred speech and dilated pupils. In younger people a body temperature of 97.6 F (36.4 C), especially when it occurs in the morning and does not rise during the day, can be an early sign of thyroid disease. Repeated lower-than-normal body temperatures warrant a medical consultation; a temperature of 97 F or less in an elderly person warrants medical attention.

BREAST SELF-EXAMINATION

Most women who examine their own breasts regularly are able to notice a possible abnormality early enough to avoid drastic treatments; they also become aware that most breast lumps are not cancerous.

Breasts should be self-examined once a month. If you are menstruating, a few days after the menstrual period is the best time, since at other times of the month—especially just before menstruation—the breasts are more apt to be swollen or tender. If you examine your breasts on the same day each month, you are more likely to recognize any change. While there are several techniques for breast self-examination, once you have learned a method satisfactory to you, consistency and regularity are the key to successful testing. Some women find that bath or shower time is easiest; others prefer lying in bed. In any event, the basic steps include (Figure 47):

- Observation: stand in front of a mirror with your arms by your side, then with your hands on your hips and your elbows as far back as possible, and then with your arms straight up over your head
- Palpation: first while you are standing in front of the mirror and then while lying on your back with one arm (the arm on the same side as the breast being examined) behind your head and using the rib cage for resistance, press the fingertips gently but firmly into the breast tissue, using a circular motion from the outside in toward the nipple, until the entire breast has been palpated
- Squeezing the nipple to observe whether there is any discharge.

Women who examine their breasts regularly and detect a lump that requires treatment have less than half the need that those who never practice self-examination have for any major surgery.

There are, however, many women who find self-examination distasteful. For such women, there is a Breast Cancer Screening Indicator (BCSI), a kit consisting of two pads, worn inside a brassiere for 15 minutes, that measure temperature changes over the entire breast and indicate any suspicious areas through color changes. The test can be repeated monthly. The comparative

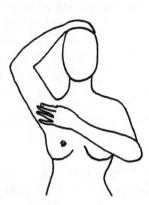

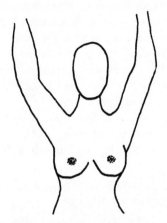

While standing, press the fingertips into the skin under the arm and then in a circular motion over the entire breast (some say that this part of the examination is more sensitive if performed when the skin is wet and soapy).

While in front of a mirror, raise both arms over your head and look for any bulges, dimples or depressions on the skin of the breasts.

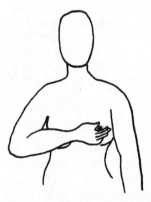

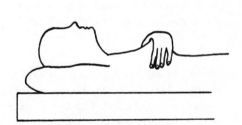

Gently squeeze the nipple to see if there is any sort of discharge or secretion.

While lying down, press the fingertips against the breast, using the underlying rib cage to provide a resistant background.

Figure 47. Breast self-examination

effectiveness of this test to breast self-examination is still under investigation.

It must be kept in mind that most breast lumps are cysts (doctors call them fibrocysts), and about one woman in five will develop one or more of these often-tender cysts between the ages of 20 and 50. These cysts are believed to be related to monthly hormone changes and usually disappear after the menopause. Recent medical advances now offer many treatments that are alternatives to surgery.

Many drugs and some foods are believed to cause breast cysts. Some women have been "cured" by avoiding certain medicines or by eliminating one or more of the following from their diets:

- Foods: those containing caffeine, such as coffee, tea, cocoa and some cola drinks; foods (chicken, beef) that contain residual traces of hormones fed to animals may cause breast swelling
- The excessive use of vitamin E has also been followed by breast cysts in some women
  Nonprescription medicines: those containing caffeine or a methylxanthine, such as Anacin, Dexatrim, Dristan, Empirin, Excedrin, Midol, NoDoz; many pain relievers, cold and sinus preparations, and appetite suppressants
- Prescription drugs, especially those containing theophylline, used to treat asthma and other chest conditions, and pain relievers that include methylxanthine products
- Hormones: birth control pills (although some women find that their cysts disappear when taking oral contraceptives); estrogens after the menopause.

Your doctor or pharmacist can tell you if any of the above-mentioned ingredients are found in your medicine.

What Is Usual

When you stand in front of a mirror, you may notice that one breast is slightly different from the other; this can be in size, shape or even position (one slightly higher than the other). This can be quite normal and once you become aware of these differences, they will cause no apprehension. While you are palpating, the tissue should be of the same consistency in all areas (it is not unusual for the tissue in the lower half of the breast to seem a little firmer to the touch than that of the upper half, but it will still be of an even consistency). Upon squeezing the nipple, there should be no discharge. When wearing the heat-detecting pads in a brassiere, there should be no "hot spots," or areas of different temperatures.

What You Need
The test primarily requires patience and the willingness to spent 15 minutes one day a month to perform the examination properly. Should you be reluctant, have your sexual partner perform the examination, doctors frequently teach husbands and partners the proper technique. The brassiere pads are sold by Fabergé at a cost of $10.00 for two sets (the extra pair is for retesting, should there be some question as to the apparent results).

What to Watch Out For
The major stumbling blocks are fear and apprehension, allowing unfounded suspicions to prevent a proper examination, an unwillingness to acknowledge the finding of what seems to be a lump and an even greater unwillingness to seek professional diagnostic follow-up. If you are not sure of how to perform breast self-examination properly, have your doctor show you and review your technique. Be sure to learn whether any medicine you are using contains any form of methylxanthine (caffeine is but one form).

What the Test Results Can Mean
The suspicion or finding of any lump in the breast warrants further testing by a physician. This could include:

- Simple observation on a monthly basis
- Mammography (special X-rays)
- Aspiration (an office procedure in which the doctors withdraws fluid or tissue for further examination)
- Biopsy (removal of a small piece of the lump for further examination).

Any wrinkling or dimpling of the skin over the breast, a discharge of any kind from the nipple, any color differences seen in the heat-sensitive breast pads or, in fact, any change—no matter how subtle—from what had been usual warrants medical attention.

Note: A recent psychological survey revealed that women who regularly examine their breasts tend to have a high self–esteem, less anxiety and more comfortable relationships with other people than women who do not; they also are known to take more responsibility for their own health.

DENTAL PLAQUE DISCLOSURE

Tooth plaques are really colonies of bacteria. They secrete two substances: a gluelike material that allows them to adhere to the surface of the teeth and an enzyme that breaks down complex sugars and white flour, causing acid to be produced. It is the acid that can erode the tooth's surface (enamel) and also dissolve the calcium that comprises the hard tooth substance. The end result is, of course, a cavity. Once plaques are established, and ignored, they can last for years and continually damage the teeth. They also contribute to periodontal disease: gingivitis, or infection of the gums, and pyorrhea, or an infection of all the tissues around the teeth, which can destroy the bones that hold the teeth in place, causing the teeth to rot and fall out. After a while plaques can turn into tartar, the whitish, hard bits of plasterlike material whose rough surface can cause bleeding gums and loose teeth.

Prevention of the initial plaque formation can be the most effective means of preventing tooth decay and the eventual need for dentures. Plaque prevention really involves proper cleaning of the teeth and gums—not simply brushing, but using the right toothbrush (with small enough bristles); cleaning between the teeth with dental floss; and adequate irrigation of the teeth and gums to remove the plaque and food particles after they have been loosened. The success of regular preventive tooth care can then be tested by the application of disclosing substances, which will reveal any remaining plaque.

What Is Usual
Plaques in their natural state are virtually invisible to the naked eye—even on close inspection. Most home plaque-disclosing preparations consist of tablets or solutions of erythrosine—the federal government's approved FD&C (Food, Drug and Cosmetic) red No. 3 dye. When a tablet is chewed, or a solution is rinsed throughout the mouth, plaque will usually show up as a vivid dark red color against a pink background (Figure 48). Obviously, no evidence of any dark red stain on or adjacent to the teeth is normal, albeit absence of such staining is not always usual. And the tongue and parts of the gums may also seem to absorb some of the stain, giving a false impression of plaque.

What You Need
The test requires disclosing tablets, such as Butler's Instant Red-Cote, which costs $4.00 for a package of 125 tablets; most dentists will give their patients,

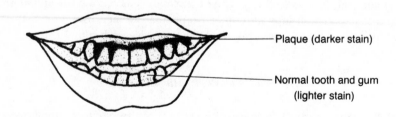

Plaque (darker stain)

Normal tooth and gum
(lighter stain)

Figure 48. Dental plaque detection.

without charge, sample packages of four tablets for home use. Packages of 1,000 cost less than $10.00 (you only use one at a time). Several other companies make disclosing tablets at similar costs. Disclosing solutions, such as Sultan, cost $1.50 for a two-ounce bottle, but you only use 10 drops at a time diluted in an ounce of water. There are many other commercial solutions, and some companies combine the discloser in gels, while others incorporate it in cotton-tipped sticks.

What to Watch Out For

Do not be surprised if your whole mouth seems to turn red, especially the first time you use any plaque discloser; the color will disappear in a short while with rinsing. Many people test for plaque at bedtime, so the color will be gone by morning. If you are not sure what you see (what is stained plaque and what is not), have your dentist demonstrate the procedure for you; he or she can also show you the best way to remove your plaque. If you have a thyroid problem or know you are unusually sensitive to iodine, check with your doctor before using dental plaque disclosers that contain iodine.

What the Test Results Can Mean

Evidence of distinct dark red stains on the teeth and along the gum line usually means plaque. It also means that your tooth cleaning and mouth care are inadequate. If you can reclean your teeth, removing the red stains—especially those that go in between the teeth—using floss, you are markedly diminishing your chances for cavities. If you find that home cleaning does not seem effective, you may already have formed hard tartar, which is best removed by your dentist. You will also learn just what areas of your teeth you have usually ignored, and this alone will improve your dental hygiene. Plaque disclosure is only one means of preventing cavities; proper diet and fluoridation (depending on your geographic location and your personal beliefs) can also contribute to long-lasting teeth and a healthy mouth.

Note: Erythrosine contains iodine as part of its chemical makeup; it could affect any thyroid function tests, so be sure to tell your doctor if you are using plaque disclosers before any medical testing.

DRUG IDENTIFICATION

Have you ever taken a drug that seemed to cause an unusual side-effect such as extreme weakness, hallucinations, an inability to think clearly, profuse sweating or slurred speech? Have you ever come across a strange pill, capsule or powder in your home and wondered what the substance was? Should you suspect the possibility of dangerous street drugs such as barbiturates, cocaine, Dilaudid, heroin, Preludin or Quaaludes, to name but a few, you can now find out anonymously what the unknown drug is. Here is what to do:

- Wrap the equivalent of one dose of the drug in aluminum foil (one tablet, capsule or some of the powder)
- Place the sample in a padded envelope, along with $15 in cash or money order; you do *not* have to give your name or otherwise identify yourself with a personal check
- Label the sample with your code consisting of five numbers of your choice followed by a letter of the alphabet
- Include any information you may have as to your suspicion of what the drug might be, the city and state where it was obtained and/or used, any effects the drug caused or undesirable side-effects that you observed or were told about and the price paid for the drug, if known
- Send the sample to: Pharm-Chem Laboratories, Dept. B, 3925 Bohannon Drive, Menlo Park, CA 94025
- After three days call the laboratory at area code (415) 328–6200 (Monday through Friday), give your personal code number and the results of the analysis will be given to you
- If you do give your name, a written report of the test results will be sent to you
- *NOTE*: if you want more than one sample analyzed, you must wrap each sample separately in its own envelope and enclose $15 for each sample
- If your sample is a water-based solution that might contain a drug, you must make prearrangements with the laboratory by phone.

The laboratory will test your submitted sample for 350 different drugs and adulterants; many street drugs also contain adulterants and diluting agents that can be a greater hazard than the drug itself. They will only tell you the name of the drug, they will not tell you the quantity or strength except through a court order. The laboratory is licensed to test drugs anonymously by the Federal Drug Enforcement Administration on the condition they pass on to the agency the results of the test and where the envelope containing the drug sample was postmarked. This provides the agency generalized information about what kinds of drugs are being offered and used and where.

What Is Usual
The only usual finding is when an unknown drug turns out to be what it is supposed to be.

What You Need
Aluminum foil and a padded envelope (available in most post offices and stationery stores).

What To Watch Out For
Do not send in vitamins, food or herb samples; do not request insecticide or herbicide analysis; do not sent in blood, urine or other body excretions or

secretions. Be sure the drug effect you experienced or observed was not due to the use of alcohol alone or in combination with a drug.

What The Test Results Can Mean
The sooner illicit drug use is discovered, the easier it is to treat and the more successful the treatment is apt to be. Of interest, the laboratory reports that more than half of all drug samples submitted to it for anonymous analysis contain drugs other than those alleged. The identification of the use of a dangerous street drug, hazardous adulterant or diluting agent warrants medical attention for the user.

EDEMA

Although observation for edema may not seem, at first, to be a medical test, in point of fact it can be one of the best diagnostic discovery techniques; it is in the same category as skin, personality and weight observation. Edema means water retention—the accumulation of abnormal amounts of tissue fluids under the skin—most commonly in the face or lower extremities, within or around the lungs, around the heart, within the cranium around the brain or in the abdomen. Observing where it is located, how much seems present and whether or not it can be "pitted" can help detect its underlying cause. Pitting edema—in which, after pushing the fingertips into the swollen areas, the hollow impression of the fingers remains as a pit-type depression—usually means that at least eight to nine pounds of excess water are present.

Normally, 6 out of every 10 pounds of body weight is water, in the form of various tissue fluids. Usually, if you eat and drink as does the average person, you take in from two to three quarts of fluid a day, and your body easily rids itself of the same amount, most commonly via urine, feces, sweat and respiration. A properly working body can handle up to eight quarts of water a day without difficulty. But when the body's water-regulating system is altered or interfered with, be it by heart or circulatory troubles (varicose veins), kidney disease, liver disease, lung impairment, hormone imbalance, certain infections, allergies, anemia or simply too much sodium (salt, etc., see Miscellaneous Tests, **Salt Measurements** test) in the diet, the water is retained and usually seeks places of least resistance (particularly the skin around the eyes) or where gravity aids its storage (the feet and ankles).

Many people translate edema into puffiness, and some puffiness just cannot be helped. Hormonal changes with premenstrual tension can cause generalized puffiness regularly, even to the point where the eyeballs swell sufficiently to prevent the wearing of contact lenses. Due to anxiety or other stressful conditions, the body can produce an antidiuretic hormone, which causes retention of sufficient fluid to result in the edema. The use of many drugs, especially birth control pills and other hormones, can cause edema as a side effect, as can menopause and pregnancy. Eating meat or poultry that has been fed or injected with hormones to increase the animal's weight can cause a similar weight increase in people due to hormonally caused water retention. Taking large amounts of vitamin E can cause generalized skin and breast swelling; many plastic surgeons will not operate on a patient until the patient stops taking all vitamin E for a month prior to surgery. Eating in restaurants where foods often contain large amounts of sodium products (such as flavor enhancers, chemical dips and sprays that act cosmetically to keep lettuce green, meat red and eliminate odor from fish) in addition to excessive amounts of salt can cause a temporary bout of edema. Traveling that entails long periods of uninterrupted sitting, high altitudes or hot, moist climates can bring on edema, most often in the lower extremities. Then there is "idiopathic" edema, which seems to be unexplainable.

Recent surveys indicate that three out of every four patients who consult a physician have some form and degree of edema. It is considered the exception to the rule when a woman between the ages of 12 and 50 does not have several episodes of edema just prior to a menstrual period. And it is estimated that half of all men who visit a doctor will have some edema, if it is deliberately searched for. But the evident edema is only the tip of the iceberg; the physical and psychological symptoms edema can cause are the real problem: headaches; personality changes; difficulty in breathing; fatigue; weakness; palpitations; diarrhea; ulcerations; itching; and aches, cramps and pains, usually limited to the swollen areas. Edema, then, is not a disease but more a reflection of some underlying reaction and/or pathology; when measured for degree, location and consequence, it can be a helpful test in offering early warning signs of impaired body function, disease and psychological disorders.

What Is Usual
Any amount of edema or puffiness is really not normal, but when considered as a temporary, brief, expected response to certain body functions or environmental factors—menstruation, prolonged sitting, tight clothing (especially garters), climate change, drug use, stress or the sudden, extremely high intake of sodium—it is not necessarily abnormal. A small amount of facial edema, especially around the eyes, usually occurs after lying down for a prolonged time. Water retention that amounts to a weight gain of no more than one to two pounds in a day, lasting no more than a day or two, may also be a physiological response to some environmental precipitating factor and still not be abnormal.

What You Need
The test requires a critical eye for honest observation, a willingness to admit to puffiness and a good scale for daily weight checks.

What to Watch Out For
You should not attempt to fool yourself or unknowingly be fooled because of your diet. One medium-sized dill pickle contains 2,000 milligrams (mg) of sodium (about 10 times the amount you need all day); eight ounces of a canned vegetable, two four-inch round pancakes from a commercial mix, two hot dogs, four slices of bologna, one cup of bran, a cup of sauerkraut and just two teaspoons of baking powder all contain 1,000 mg of sodium. One hamburger or piece of fried chicken from an animal that has been fed hormones can act on the body as if it contained well over 1,000 mg of sodium. If you are hypersensitive to sodium, it only takes 1,000 mg to cause temporary edema. Check with your doctor or pharmacist to see if any drugs you are taking contain large amounts of sodium (antacids, aspirin–like products) or if they contain hormones that could cause water retention. Asthmatics taking steroid drugs usually have some edema from their medicine.

What the Test Results Can Mean
If there is no ready explanation for edema with a weight gain of more than two pounds, no matter where it appears, and especially if it lasts for more than a day, medical consultation is warranted. As a rule of thumb, severe ankle edema usually comes from heart problems; profuse facial edema most often represents kidney disease; and abdominal edema usually comes from liver disease. Pitting edema warrants medical attention even if you think you know the cause; it usually indicates far too much water retention to have come from extraneous or environmental causes or as an expected reaction to body activities. An edema that develops slowly, over a period of days, often accompanied by a slight fever, can indicate a parasitic infestation—especially trichinosis (or filariasis, if you have traveled to one of the tropical countries where elephantiasis is endemic), but it can also signal a nutritional disorder or a vitamin B_1 deficiency. Persistent puffiness of the face, especially the eyelids, and hands is an early warning sign of thyroid disease. Any edema that cannot be easily explained, especially if it lasts for more than a day or two, warrants a medical consultation.

HAIR OBSERVATIONS AND MINERAL ANALYSIS

Hair observations include:

- Presence or absence of hair
- Location (whether hair is present in appropriate or inappropriate areas)
- Areas of baldness (male or female patterns)
- Texture
- Whether or not hair can be pulled out of the scalp easily

• Shape and structure of hair roots (anagen-telogen test).

Through such observations many cases of hair loss, as well as some under-lying disease conditions, can be explained.

Hair usually grows in three stages: The anagen stage, which lasts anywhere from six months to six years, is the newly formed, growing hair; the catagen stage is the point at which hair stops growing momentarily but could start again; and the telogen stage is that in which hair stops growing completely and is most susceptible to falling out—either from physical actions such as brushing, rough cosmetic treatments or because a new hair has started grow-ing in the same place (follicle). When hair first grows, especially in children, it is usually fine and silky, without a surrounding capsule or sheath. In later life, after hair has been growing a while, it should become more coarse and curly; it also acquires color and a surrounding capsule that gives it more body and firmness. Even later in life, hair may lose its pigmentation and become gray, white or colorless.

An abnormally large growth of hair, especially in areas of the body where it would not be likely, is called *hirsutism*; the word most often refers to women who have hair growing on the upper lip, chin, chest and lower abdomen. In contrast, loss of hair, or baldness, in body areas where hair normally should be is called *alopecia*. Either of these conditions can be, but is not always, a significant signal of something being wrong.

Hair mineral analysis. Although the actual analysis of minerals in and on hair is not performed at home, the collection of the hair sample for testing is. Some laboratories request that a doctor send them hair samples, but there are hair analysis laboratories that will test hair samples submitted directly by individuals. At the present time, hair analysis is considered useful only as an aid in screening for the possibility of poisoning from toxic heavy metals: alu-minum, arsenic, beryllium, cadmium, lead and mercury. Heroin, morphine and other opiate drugs can be detected in hair for months after they were last used. As for measuring the content of mineral substances related to nu-trition or to drug use, hair analysis is still considered to be in the experimental stage.

It is believed that, as hair is formed in its follicle, it includes, as part of its protein substance, a trace of those minerals circulating in the bloodstream. Later, as hair grows, it can also include on its surface evidence of minerals in the environment (cadmium, lead, mercury) or residue from substances used on or in contact with the hair (hair dyes, shampoo, swimming pool chemicals). Thus, knowing the rate of growth of hair and exactly how far from the skin surface it was obtained may offer an additional clue as to when toxic expo-sure, if present, took place (on the average, scalp hair will grow approxi-mately one-half inch from the skin surface in four to six weeks). Some doctors feel that hair analysis can reflect exposure to toxic metals that took place months ago; blood and urine testing usually show the minerals present only at the time of testing.

Although hair from anywhere on the body can be tested for its mineral content, most hair analysis laboratories prefer hair from the nape, or back, of the neck (midway between the ears). The hair should be cut off close to the scalp; this location also helps preclude obvious public evidence of hair loss. You will need about one-half gram of hair, and this usually amounts to a scalp area that could be covered by a nickel. Most laboratories include a makeshift paper balance-beam scale to indicate the necessary amount when they send you directions and cost information. If, however, that hair has been exposed to chemicals such as permanent wave lotions, bleach, dyes, conditioning or dandruff shampoos, detergent soaps, etc., or has been subjected to physical stress from hair dryers, sunlight, swimming, etc., some of these factors, while interfering with chemical analysis, can sometimes be taken into account beforehand and allowed for in the analysis. In most such instances, however, pubic hair or other body hair becomes a better source for testing.

Hair analysis screening has been used in surveys of children for lead and other heavy metal poisoning, especially when there is a sudden falling off of learning abilities (see Brain and Nervous System Tests, **Mental Ability and Personality Testing**). It can also be of value where symptoms of depression, lethargy, irritability, hallucinations and inappropriate behavior cannot be explained by usual diagnostic studies; many of these symptoms can be the first reflection of lead or mercury intoxication. Cadmium poisoning, while related to cigarette smoking as well as to industrial exposure, is also known to cause high blood pressure when the metal accumulates in the kidneys; the first hint of cadmium toxicity could come from hair mineral analysis.

Hair loss. Hair growth, hair loss and hair pattern distribution can also be affected by drugs as well as disease. Large doses of aspirin or vitamin A, many drugs used to treat tumors, anesthetics, anticoagulant medicines and certain hormones can cause hair loss; the sudden stopping of birth control pills is a known cause of temporary baldness in women. In contrast, other drugs such as male hormones and some diuretic preparations can cause excessive hair growth—usually in inappropriate areas. X–rays, especially to the face, head or neck, can cause hair loss. And emotional stress or anxiety is a known cause of a type of alopecia that is usually reversible once the cause of the mental anguish is eliminated. A "normal" temporary hair loss can occur for two to six weeks after having a baby or following an injury.

The anagen-telogen test. When performing the anagen-telogen test, count out 10 adjacent hairs, preferably on top of the scalp, and pull at them gently; no more than 2 should come out easily, and these should look like "club," or telogen, hairs—when examined under a pocket microscope, the root at the end of these hairs should be of a ball or pea shape (clublike), with little or no surrounding capsule. The second part of the test is to count out 20 adjacent

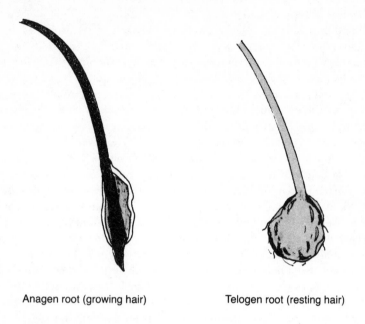

Anagen root (growing hair)   Telogen root (resting hair)

Figure 49. Hair strands and their roots after being plucked from the scalp—the anagen-telogen distinction.

hairs and, with a firm grip near the scalp, pluck all of them out; no more than 4 should be telogen hairs, while the others should be anagen hairs with the root structure at the end of the hairs more elongated, with a definite capsule or sheath around it—somewhat resembling a spear (Figure 49).

What Is Usual
Most people are quite aware of normal hair distribution; the unusual presence or absence of hair, especially if on inappropriate areas, is generally conspicuous. Depending on certain inherited traits, one can have a great deal more hair than would seem usual but still not have hirsutism; baldness, too, may be a genetic trait, and such tendencies must always be considered before labeling a "different" hair pattern as abnormal. As to texture and color, most body and scalp hair should have some pigment and firmness; it should not all be fine and colorless. As for the hair's toxic mineral content, today's environment is such that a bare trace of such minerals might be detected (less

than one or two parts per million), and while this is still not normal, it can be considered usual.

What You Need

Mostly, the test requires your powers of careful observation, combined with knowledge of your family background on hair proclivity and baldness, along with a pocket light microscope from 10-power to 30-power, which costs from $10.00 to $20.00. Hair testing laboratories can usually be found in the "Yellow Pages" under Laboratories, Medical, Research or Testing.

What to Watch Out For

You should not erroneously assume that unusual amounts of hair and seemingly inappropriate distribution are always signs of something being wrong; it could be natural for you, or it could also be idiopathic, meaning a specific diagnosis cannot be made but is most apt to be genetic. If you are suffering from dandruff (seborrheic dermatitis), acne, or a bacterial or fungus infection of the scalp, or if you have been applying any sort of chemical to the scalp (dyes, permanent wave solutions, excessive heat or even unusual hair tonics), you must clear up the underlying condition or avoid the chemicals for several months before you can use your hair for test purposes. If you suffer from trichotillomania (a condition in which a person constantly pulls hair out in either small or large amounts), this, while not a hair condition per se, warrants a medical consultation before proper hair testing can be performed.

What the Test Results Can Mean

Hirsutism, or excessive hair, especially in the wrong places on a woman, most often signals a tumor, usually in the adrenal gland, the ovary or the pituitary gland. Some examples include chest and chin hair, along with pubic hair growing up to the umbilicus, as it does in men (a woman's pubic hair usually stops growing in a straight line across the lower abdomen well below the umbilicus). Hyperactive glands without tumors can also cause hirsutism. Profuse abnormal hair growth warrants medical attention.

Baldness, or hair loss, is most often hereditary, as is the age when it becomes noticeable. Inherited male pattern baldness usually starts with a receding hairline at the forehead and proceeds along the top of the head; hair along the sides behind the ears and in the eyebrows rarely falls out. Female hair loss occurs over the entire scalp (including the sides), but it is more apt to be of a thinning type rather than a total hair loss as with men; it can also be a normal consequence of aging or the after–effects of traumatic hair treatment. Patchy, thinning hair loss in a few separated areas and unrelated to drug use is most often associated with a scalp infection; when the patches show complete loss of hair, leaving distinct circular areas of baldness, it could be an inherited trait or the result of an emotional problem, but it could also be the consequence of thyroid or parathyroid disease, old infections (syphilis, fungus), toxic metal exposure, anemia or psoriasis. Any unexplainable loss of hair warrants a medical consultation.

If the anagen-telogen test shows more than 3 telogen-root hairs out of 10, it most likely reflects a drug effect, a recent illness, pregnancy or emotional stress, and the hair will often regrow once the underlying condition is resolved. If all the hairs show anagen-type roots, or if hairs that seem to fall out on their own are of the anagen type, and drugs cannot be blamed, a medical consultation is warranted to search for the underlying cause.

Any hair mineral analysis that shows abnormal levels of toxic minerals should first be repeated—preferably at a different laboratory. In one instance, when hair was taken from one individual, divided into two equal test samples and sent to two different hair analysis laboratories, almost totally opposite results came back. Consistently reported high levels of toxic metals in hair—especially in children who show possibly related symptoms—warrant a medical consultation and confirmation by other, more specific, tests.

RADIATION MONITORING

Exposure to radiation or radioactivity can be extremely dangerous to your health. The sources of possible exposure include:

- Nuclear power plants
- Testing of nuclear weapons
- X-rays and radioactive chemicals for medical diagnosis and treatment
- Disposal of radioactive or nuclear wastes
- Microwave ovens
- Radio and television transmission waves
- Old television receiving sets (especially color sets manufactured prior to 1970)
- Jewelry made with radioactive metals (old gold and some irradiated blue sapphires from Africa; ceramic and cloisonné types from Taiwan)
- Irradiation of feeds (for sterilization and preservation)
- Some smoke detectors
- Some static eliminators used to treat film and phonograph records
- Pottery glazed with uranium oxides (usually colored orange or red); some kitchen and bathroom tiles made immediately after World War II
- Old clocks and watches painted with luminous radium
- Some camping lanterns
- Cigarette smoke

- The atmosphere (from cosmic radiation and radioactive material in the ground)
- Old buildings (constructed with radioactive materials).

The damage that can occur in your body from exposure even to only very slight amounts of radioactivity is such that there is sufficient reason to measure your environment constantly to detect how much radiation you are being exposed to and how much of that radiation your body absorbs.

There are two basic kinds of radiation: ionizing and non–ionizing. Ionizing radiation comes from X-ray machines, radioactive chemicals, nuclear generators and weapons, and "background" (cosmic radiation, from the sun and atmosphere; and earthly radiation, from radioactive material in the ground, in water and even in some foods, all acquired from naturally occurring radioactive substances such as uranium).

Ionizing radiation refers to that form of radioactivity which in very minute amounts can ionize, or break down and destroy, the cells that make up body tissues. Ionizing rays are usually described as alpha, beta and gamma. Alpha rays can be stopped by a piece of paper and are usually not harmful unless they get inside the body, where they are extremely dangerous. Beta rays can cause skin burns and internal damage but can usually be stopped by a thin sheet of metal. Gamma rays are high-energy penetrating rays such as X-rays and nuclear radiation (as from a bomb), which can only be stopped by very dense shielding, such as thick layers of concrete and lead. All three types of rays are usually emitted at the same time and from the same source, but cosmic radiation consists mostly of alpha and beta rays.

Ionizing radiation may be recorded in different ways. The basic measurement unit is the *Roentgen*, abbreviated as *R*, which indicates the amount of radioactivity being emitted by the source (an X-ray machine, a nuclear weapon, etc.). Usually, unless measuring an accumulative dose, R is measured in relation to time and is recorded as R per hour. But because radioactive emissions are most often much smaller than 1 R, they are most commonly reported as milliRoentgens per hour, or mR per hour (R = 1,000 mR).

When calculating the amount of radioactivity the body absorbs, the unit of measurement is the *rad* (radiation *a*bsorbed *d*ose); in general, direct exposure to 1 R of gamma rays, such as X–rays, results in the body's receiving and absorbing 1 rad. A third term, used mostly in medicine, is the *rem* (radiation dose *e*quivalent in *m*an), which reflects the estimated biological effect or damage of the radiation absorbed dose, or rad. A rem takes into account the damaging effect of the different kinds of rays (alpha rays once ingested or inhaled can cause 10 times as much tissue damage as gamma or X rays).

Whether or not radiation causes damage depends on several other factors: the distance from the source of the rays; physical obstacles in the way of the rays, such as clothing or protective shielding; whether the source of the radioactivity is performing properly (a correctly calibrated X-ray machine); and whether radioactive material is ingested, inhaled or injected.

A few examples: A single chest X-ray, taken with the machine six feet away, depending upon the technician's skill, can cause the body to absorb from 0.05 to 25 rads (sometimes expressed as 50 to 25,000 millirads; 1 rad = 1,000 millirads). A G-I (gastrointestinal) series, in which the esophagus, stomach and small intestine are fluoroscoped and X-rayed continually, can cause the body to absorb from four to six rads each minute the test is conducted (usually from 10 to 20 minutes). And it is not unusual for some medical diagnostic procedures such as cardiac catheterizations to cause body absorption of from 50 to 100 rads each time. The use of radioactive iodine to treat hyperthyroidism can deliver 5,000 to 10,000 rads.

A recent congressional report on X-ray exposure concluded that the greatest source of excessive, dangerous radiation is unnecessary X-ray examinations, most often performed by unskilled and untrained technicians using poorly maintained equipment. As but one example, more than 4 million gastrointestinal series are performed in the United States every year—more as a routine procedure than as a specific diagnostic test. And 75 percent of all non–hospital X–rays in the United States are taken by doctors and technicians who have not had specialty training in the science of radiant energy and its effects. These non–radiologists who own their own X-ray machine perform twice as many X-ray examinations as radiology specialists.

Governmental and scientific studies indicate that individuals over 18 years of age should not be exposed to more than 300 mR (0.3 R) a week and not more than a total of 5 R a year. After the age of 18, there is a formula to indicate excessive radiation exposure: Using 5 R as the maximum, simply subtract 18 from your age and multiply by 5. Thus, by the time you reach the age of 19, your total cumulative exposure since birth should not have exceeded 5 R. By age 30 it should be no more than 60 R, and by age 50, no more than 160 R. These figures could also be measured as rads. Children under the age of 18 should not be exposed to more than 100 mR per year. Of interest, some color television sets manufactured before 1970 can emit an average of 2.7 mR per hour at the screen's surface. A child regularly using that television set as part of a video game or computer screen can, while close to the screen, have an eye and thyroid gland radiation biological effect of from 800 to 900 millirem (mrem) per year (1 rem = 1,000 mrem).

Some other consequences of radiation: exposure of a fetus to only 1 R during pregnancy increases by 50 percent the child's chance of having cancer before reaching the age of 12; from 2 to 5 R can cause malformation of a fetus and chromosome damage; 50 accumulated R can double one's chances of having leukemia; 200 R can stop sperm production in a man and menstruation in a woman; 400 R can be fatal, although death may not occur until months later. All ionizing radiation is accumulative; small doses over a period of time can add up to a damaging amount.

Other sources of ionizing radiation include gold rings and jewelry contaminated with radioactive material. Gold that had once been used to treat cancers was subsequently recycled and used by 30 to 40 jewelry manufacturers in the making of jewelry. People who purchased jewelry made from this recycled gold have since been treated for dermatitis and skin cancers, necessitating skin grafts and amputation of ring fingers. Radiation has even been detected in cigarette smoke, and this radioactive smoke can be inhaled by nonsmokers in the same room; it has been linked to lung cancer. Smoking 1½ packs of cigarettes a day for a year is equivalent to the same radioactivity exposure of 300 chest X-rays.

Radiation sickness, most often from exposure to excessive diagnostic or therapeutic X-rays, can cause extreme weakness; loss of appetite; nausea; vomiting; hair loss; pigmentation and atrophy of the skin and dilated blood vessels on the skin, similar to spider angioma (see Miscellaneous Tests, **Skin Observations**). These consequences are not always permanently damaging, and most disappear after treatment.

Radiation damage from ionizing radiation injures the body by interfering with its ability to manufacture blood cells and by destroying the walls of blood vessels and the lining of the intestinal tract, causing severe anemia; an inability to fight off infections and cancers; an inadequate blood supply to the brain and spinal cord; and swelling, ulceration and hemorrhage of the stomach and intestines. It has been postulated that up to 3 percent of all cancers come from cosmic radiation.

Damage from ionizing radiation affects various body organs and tissues quite differently (the breast and thyroid gland are far more sensitive and more easily damaged than the kidney or brain), and any organ damage may not become evident for several hours to several years after exposure.

Non-ionizing radiation comes from some radio and television antennas, microwave generators and ultrasound devices and can be less harmful that ionizing radiation. Non-ionizing radiation requires a much greater amount of exposure than ionizing radiation before damage is seen (a diathermy machine could damage tissue if allowed to produce excessive heat). Damage from non-ionizing radiation usually shows itself at the time of exposure.

With all this in mind, you should know that, although cosmic radiation in Denver, Colorado is more than twice what it is at sea level in New York City (because of high altitude Denver averages from 75 to 140 millirads; New York City averages from 15 to 35 millirads), New Yorkers still have twice the amount of cancer as do the people who live in Denver. This only serves to show how limited our knowledge of actual radiation effects still is.

What Is Usual

Although it may not seem normal, it is usual to be exposed to some cosmic and earthly radiation at all times; the amount can depend on where you live and how much structural and other shielding there is. For every 5,000-foot rise in altitude above sea level, the rate of cosmic radiation is about doubled. If you were to measure radiation on a meter, it would not be unusual to detect about 50 mR (0.05 R) when you are standing outdoors at sea level. Occasional traveling in an airplane could expose you to some additional radiation, but because of the brief periods at high altitude and some shielding from the metal fusilage, it averages only one mR (0.001R) per trip; airline personnel, however, can more than quadruple the amounts of their natural background radiation.

Depending upon your work, you could be exposed to three or four times more radiation than in your nonwork environment, especially if you work with X-rays, nuclear chemicals and other electronic equipment, or near nuclear test sites. Radiation from medical, dental and industrial sources is not considered a usual exposure, albeit it may be helpful or necessary.

What You Need

The test requires a radiation detection device; such devices are sold under many different names: dosimeter, home or personal Geiger counter, radiation alert monitor, radiation contamination detector, radiation meter, radiation survey meter. They can come with the ability to test for radiation exposure in various ranges—anywhere from 0 to 600 R (some show how many mR strike you per hour). Most personal dosimeters are calibrated in mR (one-thousandth of an R) and go to 1,000 mR. They usually measure and total the accumulative radiation exposure while being used. Area radiation detectors commonly have both low and high ranges from 0 to 50 mR per hour; they indicate momentary exposure but do not total the dose. Most meters test for all three types of ionizing radiation, but there are meters that are limited to only one form, should you want to limit testing to food or your pet fish bowl water. Dosimeters are usually worn on the body (similar to a fountain pen) and have optical gauges that can be read in a way that resembles how one looks through a telescope; they are considered the most accurate and are used for medical-legal purposes; doctors, nurses and technicians who use X-rays wear them. They also usually require separate chargers to reset them back to zero for reuse. Geiger counters or radiation alert monitors are hand-held, pocket-book-sized instruments that have direct-reading number gauges, digital displays and colored lights to indicate various ranges of immediate radioactivity translated to what would be an hourly exposure; some also have light and sound alarms that can be preset to go off when a specified amount of radiation is detected.

There are so many different monitors available that it would be impossible to list them all; suffice it to say that they range in price from $60.00 to $90.00 for a dosimeter (plus $90.00 for a charger to reset it back to zero) and from $69.00 to $300.00 for personal Geiger counters and general radiation exposure monitors, which can test air, water, buildings, food, etc., they do not require recharging. A tissue-equivalent dosimeter, which directly indicates how much radiation has been absorbed by the body, costs $200.00. A detector to monitor only microwaves costs about $20.00.

To protect yourself against damaging ultraviolet radiation from sunlight, there is a dosimeter called TanTimer, which costs $3.00 and can be used 10 times before replacement is required. It takes into account the type of skin (for people who burn easily or only minimally) and then signals when the maximum tanning dose of radiation has been reached.

What to Watch Out For

Try to ascertain just how much radiation you will be measuring; if you are monitoring low-range amounts (cosmic, earthly or other environmental sources, X-rays or industrial use), you do not need high-range or multirange detectors; low-range detectors usually cost less. If you want to monitor all the radioactivity you are exposed to over a selected period of time, you might prefer a dosimeter that ranges from 0 to 600 R. Be aware that while some detectors come with an on-off switch, others do not and will continuously detect any and all radioactivity, whether from an old luminous watch, television set, some building materials and all background radiation, which could distort a particular measurement. Some detectors have to be recalibrated regularly; usually the manufacturer performs this service. Before you undergo any X-ray procedure, be sure to find out if there might be some other way for your doctor to make a diagnosis, and do not request X-rays purely for your own satisfaction. It has been reported that chest fluoroscopy examinations on women have caused as much breast cancer as that suffered by Japanese women exposed to the atom bombs at Hiroshima and Nagasaki.

If you do have a radiation monitor, you might want to tie it around your waist or hold it on your lap when having medical or dental X-rays; this will indicate the protective efficiency of the lead apron you should be wearing.

What the Test Results Can Mean

Radiation monitoring can offer an early warning signal for those who are exposed to any and all forms of radioactivity. Knowing how much ionizing radiation you are subjected to, and then avoiding additional exposure, can help prevent a great deal of suffering. Evidence of continuing exposure to radiation or of exposure to excessive radiation during diagnostic procedures or therapy warrants a medical consultation even if no symptoms of radiation sickness are present.

SALT MEASUREMENTS

It would be hard to imagine that there is anyone who has not been made aware of the existence of some sort of relationship between salt (sodium) and high blood pressure. At the same time, scientific evidence linking the two is not absolutely conclusive. Still, many medical authorities now advise nearly everyone to lessen the intake of salt, as well as sodium from other sources, such as:

- The sprinkling of salt over food; studies have shown that the "typical" amount added in this way is from 100 to 150 milligrams (mg) of sodium for each food item; one teaspoon, or about 5 grams (5,000 mg), of salt contains about 2,200 mg of sodium
- Eight ounces of tap water (using an average mineral analysis of drinking water from all over the country) contains from 15 to 75 mg of sodium; chemically softened water that uses salt for recharging can contain from 50 to 200 mg for every eight ounces
- Flavor enhancers such as monosodium glutamate (MSG), disodium inosinate and disodium guanylate; food antioxidants, such as sodium meta bisulphite and sodium bicarbonate, in which foods are dipped or with which they are sprayed to keep a fresh color and disguise spoilage and odors, can add another 100 to 1,000 mg of sodium to packaged or processed foods; the ingredients usually, but not always, appear on the labels of prepared foods but are rarely revealed in restaurant foods
- Most condiments are salt-based: ketchup averages 200 mg of sodium per tablespoon, mustard 900 mg per tablespoon (French-style contains even more), and soy sauce has 1,050 mg per tablespoon
- Most canned and commercial food contains much more salt than would usually be used at home: a 10½-ounce can of Campbell's chicken noodle soup contains 2,573 mg of sodium; a 3½-ounce portion of canned tuna fish in oil averages 800 mg; and a slice of commercial bread can have 150 mg of sodium
- Most "fast-food" meals also include from 2,000 to 4,000 mg of sodium (a small hamburger on a bun with all the trimmings contains 1,000 mg)
- Many medicines contain sodium: one dose of Alka-Seltzer has 521 mg of sodium; a daily dose of some forms of penicillin tablets can contain 1,000 mg; and if vitamin C is made of sodium ascorbate instead of ascorbic acid, its sodium content is almost equal to that of table salt.

Sodium is a normal body and blood electrolyte (atoms of bicarbonates, chlorides and potassium are the other major electrolytes) and is absolutely essential to maintain the body's cell functioning, water metabolism and acid-base balance. An excess of sodium in the body tends to hold excessive water in the blood and tissues until the kidneys normally eliminate it. But it does seem that some people are more susceptible than others to the water-retaining powers of sodium. It is suspected that any overload of fluid in the blood is what raises blood pressure in those who have an unusual sensitivity (possibly inherited) to sodium. Others may react to excess body fluids with edema (see

Miscellaneous Tests, **Edema**), and it is now thought that edema around the brain provokes headaches and premenstrual tension (sodium is not the only cause of water retention; cortisone products and female hormones, either naturally produced or taken as medicine, can do the same thing).

It is estimated that the "average" person on a "typical" diet takes in about 6 grams (6,000 mg, or ⅕ of an ounce) of sodium a day, equivalent to two teaspoons of salt. It is then eliminated from the body, not only by the kidneys but also by sweating (through exercise, fever or sauna sitting), bowel movements (especially with diarrhea) and vomiting. Present public health recommendations suggest reducing one's salt intake to less than 2,000 mg a day (the body supposedly uses about 200 mg a day), but many studies have shown that unless sodium intake is less than 500 mg a day, there is little or no effect on blood pressure in susceptible people; a reduced-sodium diet can help lessen edema, however.

What Is Usual
Again, no one really knows how much sodium is absolutely essential to life; it is thought, however, that any amount over 200 mg is unnecessary and automatically eliminated. Insofar as taste discrimination goes, much depends on foods first tasted as an infant, cultural practices, where one eats and physical activity. Several years ago the Campbell Soup Company reduced the sodium content of many of its foods, especially its canned soups; sales dropped to the point where additional sodium had to be put back in order for the company to stay competitive.

What You Need
In part the test requires an innate ability to perceive the flavor of salt. But even if you think your ability to discern a salty flavor is unexcelled (see Brain and Nervous System Tests, **Taste Function** test), it is virtually impossible to determine through taste alone just how much sodium you eat regularly. In one medical study people were asked to discriminate between chicken soup containing varying degrees of sodium products (salt, MSG, etc.); even those who thought they had the greatest threshold for salt discrimination and needed the least amount succumbed to selecting the soup with the greatest amount of sodium as the best-tasting. And although some food companies are now showing the sodium content on their labels, you still need a bit of mathematical agility to translate the number into reality:

- Even when itemized, the amount of sodium is usually noted per serving portion, as determined by the company; you must then decide how much you eat in relation to the manufacturer's suggested portion (some people do not dilute canned soups as much as the directions suggest and therefore take in much more sodium than the portion amount indicates)

- In some instances, sodium is labeled as to its amount in 100 grams (a bit over 3½ ounces); you must then calculate sodium intake for the exact amount of that food that you eat
- With most fresh foods, you will just have to hazard a reasonable guess (one large stalk of celery usually contains 60 to 70 mg of sodium; half of an average-sized avocado contains 350 mg; most meats average 10 mg for each ounce, while fish averages 50 mg an ounce; and there are about 60 mg in an egg)
- Pickled or cured products are, of course, made primarily with salt and usually contain from 400 mg to 500 mg per ounce, corned beef has about 270 mg per ounce, bacon over 500 mg per ounce and smoked fish up to 2,000 mg per ounce.

If you are serious about monitoring your sodium intake, there is the Original Salt Meter, which costs $100.00 from most mail order catalogs; it will instantly tell you the amount of salt and other sodium products in any liquid or solid food (including your drinking water).

What to Watch Out For
You may have a tendency, deliberately or unconsciously, to exclude from your reckoning the salt you cannot easily calculate or measure, the salt you shake on food, the sodium that is hidden in fresh pastries from the bakery, in ice cream and other fresh dairy products, and whatever you eat away from home. But most of all, if you do want to avoid sodium, watch out for labels on foods and learn to decipher euphemisms for ingredients that masquerade as something else: flavor enhancers, "natural flavor" etc. And keep in mind that the amount of sodium in packaged foods can change periodically; over the past five years Campbell's has increased the sodium content of some of its foods from 10 percent to 40 percent.

You may also be surprised to learn that some foods labeled "low-salt," "low-sodium" or "no salt added" may still contain large amounts of sodium. This is legal labeling, even if the ingredients naturally contain large amounts of sodium; only salt added during processing must be indicated on the label.

And watch out for low-sodium products that use potassium as a substitute; too much potassium can be harmful, especially when you are taking certain medicines. Check with your doctor before you start using potassium products other than naturally in foods in your diet.

What the Test Results Can Mean
If you are unusually sensitive to sodium, the results of sodium detection, allowing a reduced sodium intake, could offer one advantage in your fight to prevent high blood pressure or assist your doctor in treating it. In turn, less sodium in your diet could help you avoid heart disease and strokes. Less salt in the diet can also reduce edema and its symptoms.

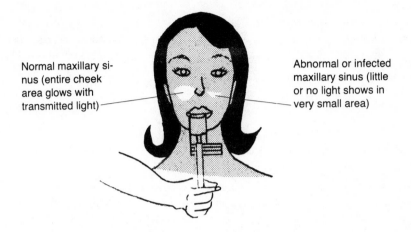

Normal maxillary sinus (entire cheek area glows with transmitted light)

Abnormal or infected maxillary sinus (little or no light shows in very small area)

Figure 50. Sinus transillumination of maxillary sinuses (the light is completely inside the mouth).

And it is very important to know that not everyone should reduce their intake of sodium. People with kidney disease and certain forms of adrenal disease; some patients with diabetes or malnutrition; those running a high fever, especially if accompanied by vomiting and diarrhea; and those who exercise or otherwise perspire profusely may be worse off with inadequate salt in the diet. Thus, it is well worth a medical consultation prior to experimenting with reducing salt in your diet. If your doctor indicates that a low-sodium diet might be helpful, then even a salt meter could be considered low-cost therapy.

SINUS TRANSILLUMINATION

Sinus problems are extremely common; what is little-known, however, is that an infected sinus can cause pains imitating dental disease, eye problems and headaches as well as chills and fever imitating serious body infections. Confirmation of a stuffed-up sinus can save much time, aggravation and money by eliminating unnecessary visits to the dentist, the eye doctor and other medical specialists. While X-rays are the definitive tests to detect occluded (blocked) sinuses, transillumination can often offer sufficient information to point out the pain-causing pathology.

Go into a darkened room and stand in front of a mirror. Place a bright light inside the mouth so that no light can be seen from around the lips when the mouth is closed. It then becomes quite easy to see if one or both maxillary sinuses (those on either side of the nose just behind the cheeks and under the eyes) are clear or cloudy (infected or congested; Figure 50). When the light

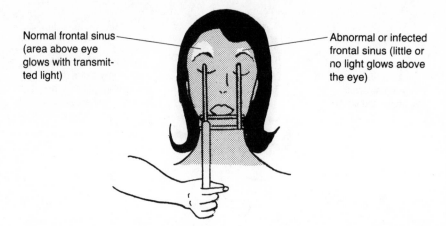

Normal frontal sinus (area above eye glows with transmitted light)

Abnormal or infected frontal sinus (little or no light glows above the eye)

Figure 51. Sinus transillumination (using a twin-transilluminator) of the frontal sinuses (the light is placed under the bony ridge just above the eye).

is placed just under the center of the bony ridge above each eye, the frontal sinuses (Figure 51) can also be checked for congestion. There are other sinuses in back of the nose, and while these cannot be checked by transillumination, they are far less frequently involved in sinusitis conditions. A bright light can also be placed in the center of each cheek, under the eyes, and the transilluminated maxillary sinuses can be viewed by looking at the palate at the roof of the mouth. Sinusitis can follow an upper respiratory infection (cold, flu) and seems much more prevalent in people with allergies. If, of course, your nose feels stuffed-up, and there is a yellowish colored mucus when you attempt to blow your nose, together with pain and/or redness over the sinus area, these factors tend to confirm sinus problems.

What Is Usual
The transmitted light should be clearly visible over each sinus area and be of equal intensity on both sides. Cloudiness or a noticeable difference in the amount of light transmitted through one or more sinuses usually indicates congestion. If you are not sure of just how much light should be visible, try the test on someone who you know has clear, open sinuses.

What You Need
The test requires a penlight-type flashlight with a very bright tip—one in which only the tip shows when it is lighted. A professional penlight made for such purposes costs from $8.00 to $12.00. A special twin-transilluminator is available with adjustable light control and twin shielded lights, adjustable for

cheek and eye width, which come together for mouth insertion; it costs from $15.00 to $20.00. These lights can also be used for transillumination of the testicles.

What to Watch Out For
Be sure the light does not show around the tip when placed against the skin or outside the mouth when the lips are closed tightly. Be sure the room is dark enough to allow transillumination to show clearly.

What the Test Results Can Mean
The cause of unexplained tooth, eye, head or face pains, when accompanied by a sinus that cannot be transilluminated, can be verified by trying nasal decongestant nose drops or sprays such as Otrivin (there are many others) to see if shrinkage and drainage of the sinus brings relief. Oral decongestants such as Sine-Off (there are many others), which work through the bloodstream, may sometimes work better than nose drops. A few drops of decongestant on a cotton-tipped stick (Q-tip) inserted gently upward in the nose for one minute is the most effective way of opening and draining sinuses. If no relief is obtained within 12 hours, and the pains persist or fever develops, a medical consultation is warranted.

SKIN INFESTATION—FLEA BITES

The three most common causes of skin infestations that are difficult to see with the naked eye (bedbugs, ticks, spiders, etc., are easily recognized) include fleas, lice and scabies (see **Skin Infestation—Pediculosis** and **Skin Infestation—Scabies**.) Once the causative insect has been identified, proper treatment can follow; more important, when the insect is known, the host factor (that is, the source of the uncomfortable dermatological condition) can be determined, isolated and treated to prevent reinfestation. The primary problem with insect bites, however, is that the red, usually swollen spots are often mistaken for other, far more serious conditions such as blood problems (purpura, see Heart and Circulation Tests, **Capillary Fragility** test), infectious diseases, allergy and eczema. Flea bites are much more common than is generally believed. And if the bites do persist and then become infected, the condition can become dangerous and quite difficult to treat.

Fleas live mostly on animals, and while household pets may be carriers, fleas are primarily found on rats, birds, chickens and especially in sandy soil, as at beaches. They obtain their nourishment by burrowing under the skin and sucking blood and are not particular—dog fleas will relish people as much as animals. Fleas also carry and transmit diseases such as plague, typhus and

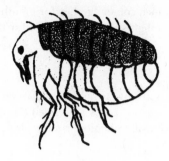

Figure 52. The flea.

even tapeworms. Although flea bites are usually more common on the lower legs, feet and exposed areas of the arms, they can occur anywhere on the body.

What Is Usual
No evidence of fleas or flea bites is normal. But if fleas do exist, they can be identified through a magnifying glass; the particular clues are the absence of wings and the unusually large, long legs in proportion to the size of the body (Figure 52). Flea eggs are white and about the size of a small grain of salt; they are more likely to be found in bedding, upholstery, carpets and even in cracks in the floor.

What You Need
You need to keep in mind the possibility that fleas may be present and have the willingness to admit same and search for them. A good magnifying glass or a 30-power battery-operated pocket light scope (microscope), which costs from $20.00 to $30.00, is also required.

What to Watch Out For
Flea bites can persist for weeks and will seem much more severe (and less like flea bites) in people who are unusually allergic. Do not be fooled if the skin shows only one or two bites; they could still be flea bites.

What the Test Results Can Mean
If you specifically identify fleas, and no infection is evident, ointments containing antihistamines or cortisone products will offer relief while you eliminate the source; through thorough washing, vacuuming and disinfection of pets, infested people, clothing and furniture. If the bites persist after a day or two of locally applied treatment, medical attention may be warranted to remove the imbedded fleas. A medical consultation may be warranted to obtain antihistaminic or analgesic medicines if the discomfort persists. Should flea bites occur while you are camping out in the woods or other remote

locations, be on the alert for a fever, rash, bronchitis or swelling under the armpit or in the groin developing anywhere from 2 to 10 days after you were bitten; this could be the first signs of plague. In fact, flea bites associated with such environmental exposure warrant medical attention to obtain preventive treatment. If spots that appear to be from flea bites persist, and no fleas or other insects are identified, medical attention is warranted.

SKIN INFESTATION—PEDICULOSIS

Pediculosis means a skin infestation of lice. It is the second of the three common parasites that can cause uncomfortable skin problems that look alike (see **Skin Infestation—Flea Bites** and **Skin Infestation—Scabies**). When statistics on lousiness were last tabulated, in 1976, more than 6 million cases of head lice infestation were uncovered in the United States, and the rate had been doubling every three years; it is now estimated that, at any given time, at least 10 million Americans are lousy. The condition is so common that any single issue of different pharmacists' trade magazines contains several full-page advertisements telling of the profit to be made by selling pediculicides and surveys showing that pharmacists supply these lice-killing medications for two out of every three cases.

Head lice (Figure 53) are but one form of the condition; there are also body lice (better known as "cooties") and pubic lice (better known as "crabs"). Body lice and head lice look similar, but the body louse is a bit bigger; all females are larger than males. Crab lice are shorter and fatter and really do resemble a crab (Figure 54); they are found mostly in pubic hair around the genitalia and in the eyebrows. Pubic lice in eyebrows and especially when in eye lashes are often misdiagnosed as conjunctivitis or infection of the eyelids; the usual antibiotic eye ointment treatment for this condition will not kill the lice and lice killing lotions are not recommended for use near the eyes. Any suspicion of lice infestation in hair adjacent to the eyes warrants medical attention. In addition, one should consider the possibility of sexual abuse to children who manifest this condition. The Public Health Service has designated pubic lice as a sexually transmitted disease. And in spite of what you may have heard, pubic lice can be caught from a contaminated toilet seat. Lice can also be picked up from theater seats—even the most expensive ones, from trying on clothing in stores, after reclaiming a coat or hat that had been checked and from a night in a hotel.

More often, though, pediculosis is transmitted by contact with someone already harboring the lice, such as schoolchildren or people who rarely change their clothes; in dormitories, barracks, camps, public transportation and queuing; and from people who share combs, brushes and clothing. As with fleas and scabies, lice are difficult to see with the naked eye, even where in-

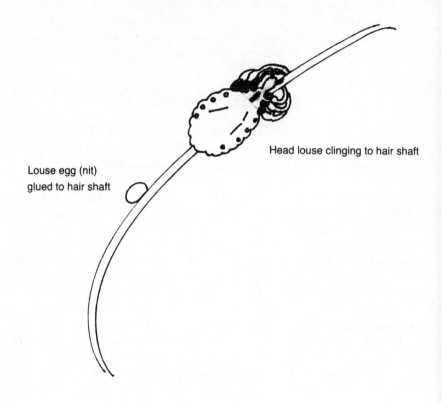

Head louse clinging to hair shaft

Louse egg (nit)
glued to hair shaft

Figure 53. Pediculosis (lice infestation)—head louse.

tense itching occurs. Usually, the first real indication of pediculosis is the spotting of a nit or several nits (Figures 53). The nits are hard, tiny, whitish gray tufts on hair strands that resemble pussy willows but are much smaller; they are the eggs, which hatch in from three to five days. The lice themselves can usually be identified through a good magnifying glass. Although lice can carry and transmit the germ that causes typhus—a serious, generalized infection that can be fatal—the primary problem is the skin infection they cause when the underlying sores are scratched and the lice feces get under the skin.

What Is Usual
No evidence of lice or nits is normal. If present, however, the nits are usually quite obvious to the naked eye. The lice may be seen after combing the hair.

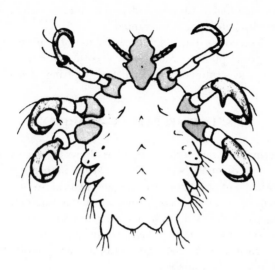

Figure 54. Pediculosis (lice infestation)—pubic louse (also called crab louse or simply "crabs"; it is found mostly in pubic hair and, inexplicably, in eyebrows).

What You Need
First you need the willingness to consider the possibility of lice infestation. A good magnifying glass or a 30-power battery-operated pocket light scope (microscope), which costs from $20.00 to $30.00, is also required.

Special disposable plastic combs that can isolate the lice and their nits, and make identification easier, called Innomed Lice-Combs are also available. These combs have beveled metal teeth that prevents scalp injury and also contain a built-in magnifier and replacable teeth so that family members cannot reinfest each other. They cost from $1.00 to $2.00.

What to Watch Out For
Mostly you should be alert for other people with obvious nits. As with so many skin conditions, pediculosis can imitate flea bites, scabies or eczema.

What the Test Results Can Mean
A specific finding of identifiable lice can be treated by several over-the-counter medications: Rid, which comes with a fine-toothed comb; A-200 Pyrinate; and Cuprex; along with sprays (Li-Ban, R & C Spray) to treat inanimate objects *only* (garments, bedding, furniture). Many of these preparations can also cause a skin reaction and must be used exactly as the directions say. They

should not be used on people with known allergies until after discussion with a doctor. If no identifiable parasite is detected and the rash or evident skin bites persist, medical attention is warranted.

Note: There is recent evidence that excessive use of nonprescription products and some prescription treatments for lice can cause nerve toxicity and blood problems; check with your doctor before applying such a medication.

SKIN INFESTATION—SCABIES

Scabies is a dermatological condition that has always been considered one of the most difficult to diagnose because the red eruption that is produced looks like so many other skin problems: flea bites and pediculosis, in particular, but it can also resemble an allergy, eczema, measles and mosquito bites—to name but a few. This particular skin infestation is reported to account for nearly 4 percent of patient visits to dermatologists in the United States. Although it occurs most often in the 15-to-45 age group, it is also found in institutions where close contact is unavoidable.

The cause is the biting of, and burrowing under the skin by, an insect called an itch mite (scientifically known as *Sarcoptes scabiei*, and more precisely an arachnid, or member of the spider family, having eight legs instead of six). The male only bites; the female both bites and burrows under the skin to lay her eggs. And it is the burrowing, most often in a corkscrew fashion, that can sometimes be observed as a clue to the diagnosis. The parasites themselves usually cannot be seen with the naked eye other than as white or grey specks.

The burrows cause itching, more frequently at night, and are most commonly found along the side of the fingers (Figure 55), on the palm side of the wrist, the elbows, the nipple area, the skin around the testicles (scrotum), alongside the penis and on the buttocks. The affinity these insects seem to have for the genital area has caused the Public Health Service to designate the condition as a sexually transmitted disease (as it has pubic lice, or pediculosis); indeed, it has been reported that from 60 percent to 80 percent of scabies cases come about by direct sexual transmission or by sleeping in the same bed with someone already harboring the mite.

But the primary problem is that the classic signs of the disease—the short, spiral burrows—are not always seen unless searched for deliberately. Failure to diagnose the infestation early enough can lead to serious overall skin infections and skin ulcers. (See **Skin Infestation—Flea Bites** and **Skin Infestation—Pediculosis**).

What Is Usual
Obviously, no evidence of an infestation is normal, but in the case of scabies, the corkscrew burrows are the definitive clue. Then, if you take a sharp steri-

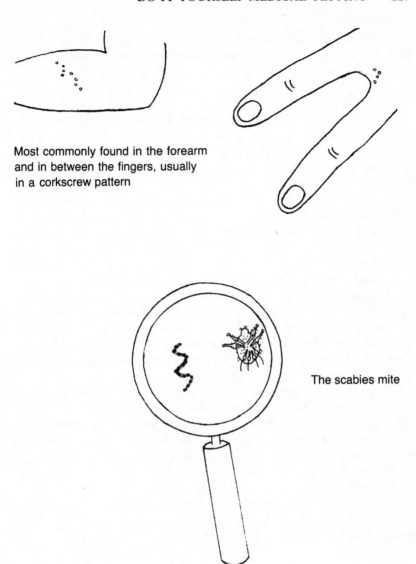

Most commonly found in the forearm
and in between the fingers, usually
in a corkscrew pattern

The scabies mite

Figure 55. Scabies infestation.

lized tweezer point (or needle or pin), dip the point into a drop of mineral
oil and probe the end of the burrow and then look at the point through a
powerful magnifying glass or through a pocket microscope, you should be
able to see the eight-legged creature or some of its dark, reddish-colored
feces.

What You Need

The test requires a good magnifying glass of at least four power, which costs from $1.00 to $10.00. A battery-operated pocket light scope (microscope), usually 30-power (magnifies 30 times), costs from $20.00 to $30.00.

What to Watch Out For

Be sure the pointed object is clean; you can hold it in the flame of a match for a second or two and then let it cool, or hold it in rubbing alcohol for a few seconds. Do not poke too hard into the end of the burrow—that is, not hard enough to draw blood. Actually, the scabies mite will cling to the mineral oil if it is merely touched.

What the Test Results Can Mean

If scabies is evident, it is quite easy to treat (the entire family should be treated at the same time). If there is no reason to suspect sexual transmission, it is important to try to locate the source to avoid reinfestation; schoolchildren have been known to bring the mites home. The discovery of the mites usually calls for nothing more than a medical consultation to obtain an effective scabicide. Should sexual transmission be possible, that medical consultation might include tests for other sexually transmitted diseases (see Genitourinary System Tests, **Gonorrhea**). Failure to detect the mites or burrows (and failure to identify flea bites or pediculosis) in the presence of any skin problem warrants medical attention—especially in very young children.

One product, A-200 Pyrinate, can be obtained without a prescription in either liquid or gel form. Although it does not claim to be a scabicide (it is primarily for the control of lice and their nits), many doctors have found it an effective treatment for scabies. Do not use this product in the presence of an infection or if you know you are allergic. And be very careful with it; do not swallow it, inhale it or allow it to come in contact with the eyes, mouth or genital areas.

Note: There is recent evidence that excessive use of non-prescription products and some prescription treatments for lice and/or scabies can cause nerve toxicity and blood problems; check with your doctor before applying such a medication.

SKIN OBSERVATIONS

Although *eczema* is the name given to any number of skin conditions characterized by redness, itching, scaling or rash, it is not a specific medical diagnosis. Beyond eczema, there are a few specific skin observations that can be early warning signs of underlying disease, and their prompt discovery and interpretation could help prevent subsequent disability. As an example: Persistent, pale-yellow-tinted, dry skin, especially when accompanied by a puffy face—particularly around the eyes—and swollen hands (see Miscellaneous Tests, **Edema**) can be the first indication of thyroid disease.

While there are many ways of describing skin changes, it will suffice to consider three basic categories:

- Color, or the presence or absence of pigment (usually does not include generalized redness)
- Physical structure: a macule is a lesion, usually colored, that is not raised above the skin surface (it cannot be felt when touched); a papule is raised above the skin surface (a tiny "bump," somewhat like a mosquito bite, can be felt); skin plaques are large papules; vesicles or bullae are blisterlike lesions containing fluid (when infected they are called pustules)
- Blanchability, or whether or not the color disappears when pressure is applied—usually by a fingertip.

The skin lesions mentioned above must be distinguished from hives, or urticaria (which differs from eczema in that it is an allergic rather than in-flammatory reaction), characterized by red, pink or sometimes pale swelling that arises suddenly and is rarely permanent (see Miscellaneous Tests, **Allergy Patch and Elimination Diet** testing); many medications can cause urti-caria, which is often precipitated or exaggerated by sunlight. Because drugs can also cause a variety of skin conditions, they must always be considered; antibiotics, aspirin and aspirinlike drugs, birth control pills, food colorings, diuretics and even some vitamins are very common causes of skin rashes.

Pigmented blemishes are most often various shades of blue, blue-red or brown (Figure 56). Dark "black-and-blue" spots (called ecchymosis) com-monly follow an injury, but if they appear anywhere on the body (petechia) without evident provocation, they can be an indication of bleeding disorders or liver disease (see Heart and Circulation Tests, **Capillary Fragility** test). If pressure is applied to these small dots, they will not turn pale or white (blanch), as do most skin lesions of no medical significance. A venous "star" appears most often on the legs; its center is a blue or purplish area about the size of a rice grain that has thin, wavy lines radiating outward one to two inches from it. They do not blanch when pressed and usually suggest the development of varicose veins. In contrast, a spider angioma is more reddish and smaller than a venous star and will blanch or momentarily disappear when pressure is applied. These usually are limited to the upper part of the body and are normal consequences of aging, although some doctors think they reflect liver problems.

The sudden appearance of brown pigmentation, especially on exposed sur-faces, can be the first indication of an adrenal disorder (Addison's disease); it can also come from anemia, cancer and several other connective tissue con-

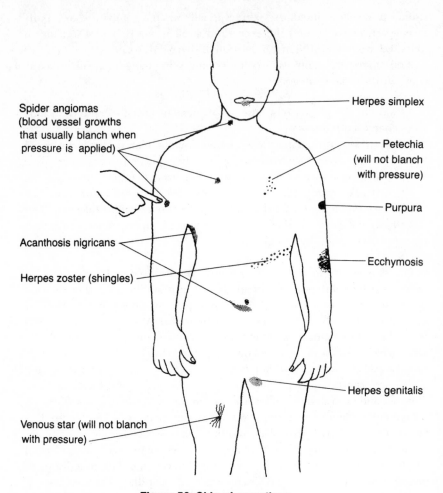

Figure 56. Skin observations.

ditions. Many women taking birth control pills also develop areas of brown pigmentation that appear most often over the cheekbones and around the nipples.

Tiny clusters or blisters appearing around the mouth, commonly called "cold sores," are usually caused by a herpes virus. It is believed that once the virus establishes itself in the body (usually in the nerves), it remains for a lifetime and can be reactivated by upper respiratory infections, sunlight and stress. The same or a different, second form of virus can also cause blisters to appear on and around the genitalia, and it has been reported that more than 20 million Americans now have genital herpes, while half a million more men and women between the ages of 18 and 35 are contracting the disease every year. It is now considered the fastest growing sexually transmitted disease in the United States. And a third form of the virus can cause blister-like lesions around the torso, following the distribution of a nerve from the spinal cord to the skin (herpes zoster, or "shingles").

What Is Usual
The skin should be clear, have good turgor (firmness and elasticity) and be free of blemishes—other than those known since birth (birthmarks). Rashes, itching, blisters, dryness, scales and any sudden appearance of lesions on the skin are not normal, albeit they may either be attributed to a drug or contact with an allergen or appear subsequent to trauma.

What You Need
The test just requires your powers of observation, applied regularly and systematically, in order to notice something new or different about the appearance of your skin.

What to Watch Out For
You must beware of ignoring a skin lesion; it may take one medical consultation, but assurance that a lesion is not serious is well worth the peace of mind it brings. Do not ignore the possible implication of any medicine you are taking; check with your doctor or pharmacist to find out which of your drugs can cause skin reactions.

What the Test Results Can Mean
Any pigmented, new skin lesion, especially one that does not blanch when pressed, warrants a medical consultation. Any brown-pigmented macular (flat) or papular (raised) lesion that seems to become darker or blacker warrants immediate medical attention.

Many cancers inside the body can reflect their existence through skin lesions. Dermatomyositis looks like a profuse, reddish macular rash that is almost always accompanied by weakness of the muscles—usually, but not always, directly under the rash; there may be much more muscle weakness than obvious skin lesions, or there may be a profuse rash all over the body with only one or two muscles affected, but muscle weakness must exist to make a diagnosis of dermatomyositis. Suspicion of this lesion warrants a medical consultation. Once the diagnosis has been made, it is known that up to 50 percent of adults with this skin-muscle condition also have cancer—most commonly in the gastrointestinal tract or lung.

Acanthosis nigricans is a brown to black-pigmented papular thickening of the skin, most often under the armpits, in the groin and on the abdomen around the umbilicus or navel—especially if the skin in that area tends to fold or flop over itself. Most people who have the lesions tend to describe them as "dirty skin" that cannot be cleaned. Doctors feel that at least half of all people who develop this skin condition also have internal cancer—most commonly in the gastrointestinal tract; suspicion of this condition warrants a medical consultation.

Herpeslike blisters, especially on or around the genitalia, warrant medical attention to ascertain the diagnosis—both to protect others from catching the disease and because, if the condition is found in a pregnant woman, it can cause brain damage and death in newborns. And herpes lesions have all too frequently been associated with cancer of the cervix and lymph cell cancers, such as leukemia.

If you have been camping out in the woods or wilderness, and there were ticks in the area, any sudden appearance of petechia or purpura warrants medical attention; it can be the first indication of Rocky Mountain spotted fever. If isolated papules and/or vesicles appear, check yourself for insect bites (see **Skin Infestations—Flea Bites, Skin Infestations—Pediculosis** and **Skin Infestations—Scabies.**)

Skin conditions that do not fit into the patterns described warrant medical consultation unless you are already aware of the cause (allergies, bacterial or fungus infections, psoriasis, etc.) The sudden disappearance of skin pigmentation, most commonly called a secondary leukoderma, is usually consequence of a previous skin disease such as psoriasis, but it can also come from thyroid disease, diabetes, certain cancers and old infections such as syphilis and leprosy. It can also be the result of exposure to certain industrial chemicals. It warrants a medical consultation.

VITAMIN C BODY LEVEL

Most animals can manufacture all the vitamin C (ascorbic acid) they need in their livers; guinea pigs and certain mammals such as horses and humans cannot and, therefore, must include a minimal amount of this vitamin in their daily diet. And, even after you ingest vitamin C—either as part of your food or as a supplemental pill, capsule or powder—its biological effect only lasts about six hours. Thus, humans need constant replenishing of this particular, very essential, vitamin. Most people know that inadequate body levels of vitamin C can cause scurvy (bleeding under the skin, bleeding and swollen gums, anemia and weakness) and many people believe more than adequate body levels can help prevent colds and possibly help fight cancer. Few people, however, seem aware of the role of this vitamin in accelerating the healing of wounds (accidental or surgical), in detoxifying certain drugs and other chemicals such as nitrites, in the formation of necessary steroid hormones, in the utilization of iron in the body, in the regulation of cholesterol metabolism, in the maintenance of normal brain activity for good mental health and particularly in the alleviating of dangerous body reactions to stressful conditions. Adequate vitamin C levels in the body are essential to deter some diseases as well as fight off existing illnesses.

It is generally agreed that children through adolescence should have at least 30 to 40 mg of vitamin C in their diet; from the mid-teens through adulthood, the recommended minimum is 60 mg a day (equivalent to the amount found in four ounces of orange juice, a large ripe tomato, a cup of shredded cabbage or a three-inch long baked potato). While some scientists question the adequacy of the recommended amount for the average person, other researchers feel much larger doses are necessary especially in the face of stressful physical and mental conditions. It has been shown that individuals do use up their body's store of vitamin C much faster when confronted by disease or distress and the resulting lowered body levels of this vitamin seem to aggravate any existing illness or anxiety thus causing a vicious cycle.

Becoming aware of your own vitamin C body levels, knowing how much vitamin C you particularly require to keep your body tissues satisfied and learning how your body's vitamin C level reacts to stressful situations could be of great value to you in maintaining good health. A simple test for all these vitamin C measurements is the lingual self-test kit where a drop of a special colored reagent solution is placed on the tongue and timed to note how quickly the color disappears. This is quite different from the measurement of vitamin C in the urine (see *Urine Tests*, Vitamin C); which is primarily to detect excessive vitamin C that can interfere with other urine tests. The failure to detect vitamin C in urine, however, could also signal a deficiency of that vitamin in the body.

What Is Usual: When the drop of colored test solution is placed on the center of the tongue, it should disappear within 15 seconds; the faster it disappears, the greater your body levels of vitamin C.

What You Need: A Vitamin C Self Test Kit available in pharmacies and some health food stores or directly from the manufacturer: Abroca, Inc., P.O. Box 5582—Maple Drive Station, Beverly Hills, CA 90210. The kit, which can perform 20 or more tests, costs $9.95.

What To Watch Out For: Follow the kit's directions carefully. Do not test on a wet or thick coated tongue, and do not test after eating, brushing your teeth or using mouthwash. Keep in mind that smoking can severely deplete your vitamin C levels, as will the use of aspirin, antibiotics, cortisone drugs and oral contraceptives. Your diet and lifestyle can also affect your vitamin C body levels, but then that is what this test may help you discover.

What The Test Results Can Mean: If it takes more than 20 seconds for the colored drop of test solution to disappear from your tongue, it could mean your diet is deficient in vitamin C; it could also mean your body does not absorb the vitamin properly or that you are undergoing a sufficiently stressful situation as to deplete your body levels of the vitamin. The test kit also includes a supply of vitamin C tablets along with directions to help determine your body's absorption rate and the effects of stress. If, after taking the prescribed amount of vitamin C in the test's directions, the time for the colored test drop to disappear does not shorten to 15 seconds or less, a medical consultation is warranted. People with alcoholism, anemia, cancer, hidden infections and a host of other conditions often have inadequate body levels of vitamin C even with an adequate amount of the vitamin in their diet.

Keep in mind that while many people can take extremely large amounts of vitamin C without any obvious untoward side effects, there are those who can have an adverse reaction to such excessive doses. There is, for example, a claimed association between large amounts of vitamin C and the formation of kidney stones in certain individuals. Before you attempt to increase your daily intake of vitamin C, you should discuss the matter with your physician to be sure you are not unusually sensitive to the vitamin.

WEIGHT OBSERVATIONS

Involuntary weight loss of a few pounds rarely seems sufficient reason for a medical consultation; in many instances the loss of a few pounds either goes unnoticed or, at times, is even appreciated. But in medicine there is a maxim that any unexplainable weight loss of more than 5 percent of one's usual body weight within a one-month time period is assumed to come from some hidden disease until proved otherwise. Studies have shown that should a 100-pound woman lose more than five pounds, or a 150-pound man lose eight pounds in a month or less, the most common cause of this sudden weight loss, if not from deliberate dieting, is cancer (see Brain and Nervous System Tests, **Taste Function** test). Secondary causes of enigmatic weight loss include: stomach ulcers (see Gastrointestinal System Tests, **String Test** and **Feces Observations**); infections (see Miscellaneous Tests, **Body Temperature**); obstructive lung diseases (see Breath and Lung Tests, **Pulmonary Function Measurements**; heart or circulation problems (see Heart and Circulation Tests, **Blood Pressure**); nerve pathology (see Brain and Nervous System Tests, **Reflex Testing** and **Sensory Testing**); hormone dysfunction; and emotional problems such as depression (see Brain and Nervous System Tests: **Beck Depression Inventory**).

On the other hand, persistent weight gain is rarely a reflection of disease; it may be genetic, or it could reflect thyroid gland or other metabolic disorders, but most often weight gain comes from eating too much and exercising too little. Surprisingly, obesity and overweight do not mean the same thing. Obesity is an excess of body fat, while overweight means having a body weight greater than that shown on standard height-weight tables. A football player may be overweight because of an excess of muscle tissue, but he is not obese. Obesity, or too much body fat in proportion to the size of one's body, can become a medical problem.

While fat deposition and distribution are related to age, they are controlled primarily by body hormones. Women usually store fat in their breasts, buttocks, hips and thighs. Men, on the other hand, most often store excess fat in and around the stomach area. Obesity as a consequence of thyroid or adrenal disease, or diabetes, tends to show up more in the face, neck and upper torso.

Standard weight tables are usually correlated to one's age, sex and inherited body build as well as height. Body build is usually a reference to the size of one's skeletal frame and is most often described as small, medium or large. The tables indicating so-called normal, or desirable, weights have been derived primarily from insurance company morbidity (sickness) and mortality (death) statistics and are purported to represent the ideal weight for healthy individuals. Times do change, though, and while it used to be believed that weighing 10 percent more or less than stipulated by the standard tables was unhealthy, now most doctors feel that the figure should be a variation of 20 percent or more from "normal" before weight alone poses any significant risk.

At the time this book went to press, a revised set of weight-height-body build tables was about to be published based on new information from the Life Insurance Medical Directors of the United States and Canada. The new tables, the first changes since 1959, are expected to show ideal weights to be 5 to 15 percent higher than the figures recommended nearly 25 years ago. But even these new figures have already incurred opposition from several medical men; however, keep in mind the words on one insurance actuary: "[Such a chart] simply advises people that if they keep to this weight, they'll have the best chance of the greatest longevity."

While weight-height-body build observations are fine for generalized health screening, there are more specific parameters for measuring the amount of body fat and muscle (protein) in relation to size and weight. These include skinfold thickness and extremity circumference and diameter measurements; when considered along with standard weight tables comparisons, they are called anthropometrics. Anthropometric measurements not only can help reveal the cause of obesity (be it disease or gluttony), but they can also help assess nutritional status—malnutrition, malabsorption of food, improper or inadequate metabolism—and identify the possible cause of previously unexplained symptoms such as anemia or depression.

Skinfold thickness. When the skin is "pinched" and pulled away from the

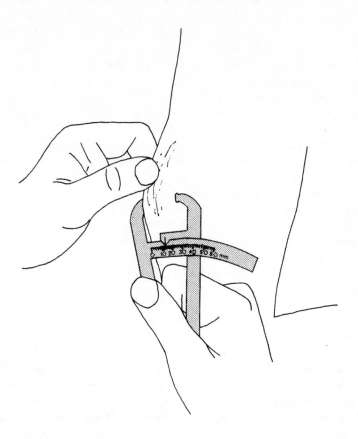

Figure 57. Using skinfold calipers (pinching the skin away from the underlying muscle and measuring its thickness; in this instance, 14mm).

body, it forms a fold, whose thickness can be measured with a caliper (Figure 57). The distance between the two skin surfaces when pulled away from any underlying muscle is considered a reasonable estimation of body fat; the amount of fat under the skin approximates the amount of fat throughout the rest of the body. While just about any skin surface can be used for skinfold thickness measurements, the two most common areas are the subscapular (just below the bottom edge of the large shoulder blade bone on either side of the back) and the triceps (the skin over the large posterior upper arm muscle, which straightens out the forearm). When performing the *triceps skinfold thickness test*, it is important to make the measurements at a standard location so that future measurements will always be at the identical place. For triceps skinfold place the upper arm at your side with the elbow bent, so that the lower arm is parallel to the floor. Measure the distance between the bony projection at the top of the shoulder and the point of the elbow, preferably in centimeters (a cloth measuring tape works best). Mark the point midway between the two bony protrusions. With the arm hanging loosely straight down at the side, at the marked point, pinch the skin and underlying fat together on the back of the arm between the thumb and index finger so that it is pulled away from the muscle. Place the jaws of a skinfold caliper around the pinched skin and muscle according to the particular caliper's directions and measure the thickness of the fold. It is suggested that three different measurements be made a few moments apart and the average of the three readings be recorded. This is considered a reasonable estimate of an individual's body fat reserves.

Extremity (midarm) circumference. Using the same point marked on the upper arm for the triceps skinfold thickness, measure the *midarm circumference*, or the distance around the arm—again, preferably in centimeters.

Midarm muscle circumference. There is a formula for estimating the body's muscle mass, or protein reserve, as opposed to fat mass. It requires you to convert your measurements to centimeters (cm) unless your tape measure is so marked (1 inch = 2.54 cm; ¼ inch = 0.64 cm). Multiply the triceps skinfold thickness in cm by 3.14 and then subtract the result from the midarm circumference measurement in cm. As an example, if the midarm circumference measured 32 cm (12½ inches) and the triceps skinfold thickness measured 12 mm (1.2 cm) by the calipers, midarm muscle circumference would be:

$$32 - (1.2 \times 3.14) = 32 - 3.77 = 28.2 \text{ cm}$$

By following the changes in weight along with arm fat and muscle measurements over a period of time, it is sometimes possible to discern the cause of weight loss or gain, especially when related to specific metabolic or digestive maladies. Such tests can also help distinguish between deliberate overeating, avoidance of food or an underlying disease.

Heatstroke sensitivity. People differ in their susceptibility to heat exhaustion or heatstroke—especially when engaged in strenuous physical activities. One particular weight observation test can help you find out how sensitive you might be to the effects of heat. Wearing as little clothing as proper, weigh yourself before and after engaging in or performing your usual sport or exercise for the usual amount of time. Perform the activity with the clothes you normally wear while being physically active. If you find you lose body water by sweating to the extent of more than 3 percent of your body weight, you are probably more sensitive than most people; if you lose more than 5 percent, you run a much greater risk of heatstroke and should be very careful, especially if your activities require clothing that causes increased sweating. And it seems the more muscular you are, the more susceptible you are to heatstroke.

What Is Usual

The figures and measurements offered in Figure 58 are compilations of several tables showing "ideal" weights; they are not meant to be absolute, as there is, at this time, no general agreement as to what normal weight should be. If your weight—according to your age, body build (Figure 59), height and sex—lies within the range of 20 percent more or less than the suggested figure, it can be considered usual. For example, the ideal weight of a 45-year-old, 68-inch-high, medium-body-framed man is listed as 150 pounds, but any weight between 120 and 180 could still be considered within usual limits.

At birth the usual weight of a child is from six to nine pounds (average 7½ pounds), and the usual length is from 19 to 21 inches (average 20 inches); the difference between boys and girls then is negligible. The rule of thumb is

Figure 58. Height=weight tables (in inches and pounds).*

	Men				**Women**		
Height	Age Group			Height	Age Group		
	18–35	36–55	Over 55		18–35	36–55	Over 55
62	125	130	130	58	100	105	110
63	129	134	133	59	103	109	110
64	132	138	138	60	105	112	115
65	135	141	141	61	108	116	117
66	138	145	144	62	111	119	120
67	140	148	147	63	114	123	123
68	145	150	148	64	118	126	126
69	149	154	150	65	121	130	130
70	154	160	155	66	125	135	134
71	158	165	161	67	130	138	137
72	162	169	163	68	134	140	139
73	165	175	164	69	138	143	142
74	170	180	172	70	142	146	145

*With indoor clothing but without shoes. Weights listed are for a medium body skeletal frame (using body skeletal frame guide—Figure 59). Those with a small frame, deduct 7 percent; those with a large frame, add 7 percent.

Figure 59. Body skeletal frame guide.

Find the two bony protrusions on either side of the wrist and, just below those points (toward the hand), measure the circumference around the wrist with a cloth measuring tape. Use the smallest measurement possible. Compare your wrist to your height, as shown below, as a reasonable indication of the size of your body build.

Height	Wrist Circumference	Skeletal Frame
Under 62 inches	Less than 14 cm From 14 to 14.5 cm Greater than 14.5 cm	Small Medium Large
From 62 to 65 inches	Less than 15 cm From 15 to 16 cm Greater than 16 cm	Small Medium Large
Over 65 inches	Less than 16 cm From 16 to 16.5 cm Greater than 16.5 cm	Small Medium Large

17 ½

that a baby's weight doubles in six months, triples at 1 year of age, and then the child adds five pounds a year until the age of 5. Growth in the first year averages about 10 inches; 5 inches during the second year; 4 inches during the third year; 3 inches during the fourth; and 2 inches through the fifth. From the age of 5 through adolescence, weight depends on inherited growth characteristics, such as height and body build, sexual development, eating habits and physical activity. The "average" boy or girl at 5 years of age is 42 inches tall and weighs 40 pounds; by 10 years they have both usually grown to 53 inches and weigh 70 pounds. By 18 years of age, the "average" boy has grown to 68 inches and weighs 143 pounds; the "average" girl is 64 inches tall and weighs 122 pounds.

During adulthood it is believed that men continue to gain weight until they reach their early forties, while women seem to gain weight until their early fifties. Weight should stay the same until the seventies, and then it usually decreases.

As for anthropometric measurements (Figure 60), usual observations show the triceps skinfold thickness and midarm muscle circumference to be within

Figure 60. Anthropometric upper arm measurements.

Age	Midarm Circumference (in cm)		Triceps Skinfold (in mm)*		Midarm Muscle Circumference (in cm)	
	Men	Women	Men	Women	Men	Women
18–19	30.1	26.2	8.5	17.5	27.4	20.7
20–24	31.0	26.5	10.0	18.0	27.9	20.8
25–34	32.0	27.8	12.0	21.0	28.2	21.2
35–44	32.7	29.2	12.0	23.0	28.9	22.0
45–54	32.1	30.3	11.0	25.0	28.7	22.5
55–64	31.7	30.2	11.0	25.0	28.3	22.4
65–74	30.7	29.9	11.0	23.0	27.2	22.7
(Should be greater than)	26.3	25.7	8.5	14.9	22.8	20.5

*If the skin behind the upper arm is pinched between the fingers, instead of using skinfold calipers, the thickness should not be greater than 12 mm (½ inch) in men and 25mm (1 inch) in women; to convert mm to cm, multiply by 10.

It is usual for women to have 50 percent more stored body fat than men; women average 22 percent body fat, while men average only 15 percent.

10 percent of the charted figures. The midarm circumference measurement can vary by 20 percent and still be usual. Much depends on whether the measurements are used to detect obesity or assess the nutritional status. In general, the triceps skinfold should not be greater than 20 mm in men and not more than 30 mm in women.

What You Need

Weight observations require a good scale—one that is accurate and easy to read. Many inexpensive scales can vary more than a pound with each use. Spring scales should have a manual zero adjustment and show weight in quarter-pounds; dial-reading scales cost from $8.00 to $20.00 where the reading is at floor level and $25.00 and up for those that show weight at waist level (this can be important if it is difficult to see around the abdomen). Digital display readout scales cost from $20.00 to $100.00, depending on where the display is located and whether or not the scale has a built-in memory factor that shows the previous weight for several members of a family. Digital scales should show weight in 0.2 pounds. Balance-beam scales (as are used in most doctors' offices) are considered most accurate, should such precision be desired, and cost from $60.00 to $200.00, depending on whether they use sets of weights on a bar or digital display to show the result; some may include a telescoping height-measurement bar. It is a good idea to check your scale at least once a month by comparing a known weight such as 25 pound-bag of kitty litter, a large box of laundry detergent or something similar.

Skinfold calipers range in cost from free to $150.00, depending on their sensitivity. For home testing, inexpensive plastic models are quite adequate. If you buy the book *Coaches' Guide to Nutrition and Weight Control*, by Dr. Patricia Eisenman and Dennis Johnson, at $9.95 (published by Human Kinetics Publishers Inc., Box 5076, Champaign, Illinois 61820), you will also receive a coupon redeemable for a free skinfold caliper along with detailed instructions on measuring body fat. One pharmaceutical company gives doctors plastic calipers at no charge, and your doctor may pass one on to you. Automotive and tool calipers, which sell for from $7.00 to $70.00, will work just as well, as will drawing calipers, which cost $4.00 to $5.00 along with a ruler marked in millimeters (mm). Precise skinfold calipers include the Lange or the Harpenden and cost from $100.00 to $150.00; they take into account skin tension, the amount of pressure applied to the instrument and even the slope of the skin surface.

What to Watch Out For

For consistency you should weigh yourself at the same time every day, preferably after awakening and having emptied your bladder. Ideally, you should wear the same garment each time. If you want to check your scales with those in your doctor's office or in a commercial establishment, be sure to wear the identical clothes each time and make the comparison within an hour's time; it is not unusual for body weight to vary one to two pounds up or down during a 24-hour period. Do not weigh yourself after a loss of body water as from exercise or diuretic pills; temporarily induced water loss usually returns within hours, and you would only be fooling yourself. The same applies to any drastic change in your diet; eating a large quantity of salty products (delicatessen food, pretzels, potato chips, etc.) can hold excess water in your body for hours (see Miscellaneous Tests, **Edema**). Many women taking birth control pills or other hormones tend to gain weight (hold water) during the first two or three weeks of their menstrual cycle. It is also possible to gain several pounds of weight after a severe emotional upset; that weight can last for up to a day or two after resolution of the problem. Be honest with yourself; if you know the cause of weight gain or loss, do not try to hide it from yourself or your doctor.

What the Test Results Can Mean

If you are more than 20 percent over or under the ideal weight suggested, a medical consultation is warranted. Even if you know you have been eating too much, or too little, such a discrepancy warrants an investigation as to the reason why. The connection between obesity and arthritis, atherosclerosis and high blood pressure, and diabetes is fairly well established, and it can make many other disabilities much worse than they would otherwise be. Obesity can be the cause, as well as the consequence, of many emotional and social problems.

An equal number of disease conditions are related to underweight. For one thing, individuals who are underweight because of malnutrition usually have very poor immunity to many other seemingly unrelated conditions, especially infections. They also fail to heal normally following an injury or surgery; they show an increased clotting time (see Blood Tests, **Bleeding and Clotting Time**), making them more susceptible to strokes; and they almost always suffer from some form of anemia (see Blood Tests, **Hemoglobin** test). As with being overweight, being underweight also causes, and results from, emotional problems, depression, irritability and memory problems seem to go hand-in-hand with malnutrition.

Any sudden weight loss in a short period of time warrants medical attention. In women of childbearing age, loss of fatty tissue can be accompanied by a loss of estrogens, or female hormones; a good portion of estrogen is stored in fatty tissue. The consequences can be menstrual irregularities—even the failure to menstruate for months at a time—and an inability to become pregnant.

Any unusual distribution of obviously excessive fat, especially when concentrated in only one or two areas, warrants a medical consultation. While obesity is not a true disease in itself, it can be an early warning sign of some other body problem. It also increases the body's work load (try carrying a 10-pound box of detergent around for a few hours). And keep in mind that edema, which rarely has anything to do with fat deposition, can also cause a marked increase in body weight; repeated bouts of edema warrant a medical consultation.

If your upper arm measurements show an excess of muscle tissue over fat (increased midarm muscle circumference over decreased triceps skinfold thickness), and your weight is much greater than predicted, it could mean your increased weight is normal for you, especially if you are an athlete or into physical fitness. If the arm measurements are reversed, however, and you are overweight, a medical consultation is warranted to rule out a hormone disorder. Should your triceps skinfold measurement be greater than usual without obesity, it also warrants a medical consultation. As you become older, and are less physically active, however, it is not unusual to show a bit more fat than muscle tissue.

Upper arm measurements that are well below usual values, no matter what your weight, warrant a medical consultation; they can be the first signs of protein malnutrition (conditions called marasmus and kwashiorkor). In elderly people anthropometric measurements that are below usual values can be clues to why certain drugs are not working as they should; they can also explain some bowel problems and prevent unnecessary surgery. In many instances the proper interpretation of upper arm measurements can point out some simple, easily correctable vitamin or mineral deficiency that can eliminate a great many uncomfortable symptoms.

Understanding the difference between overweight and obesity as well as the problems of being underweight or undernourished—and seeking professional help for any unusual weight observations—is considered one of the best ways of practicing preventive medicine.

APPENDIXES

APPENDIX I
Health Maintenance Index

Many medical tests can be performed to keep a check on the state of one's health as well as to uncover dormant diseases. Preventive medicine means more than avoiding illness; it also includes the detection of early warning signs of impending ailments, thereby permitting one to avoid or lessen subsequent disability. The following tests, when performed routinely, should help reduce the number and severity of many medical maladies. The value of many of these tests lies not so much in the individual test results as in providing a record over a period of time, so that any change can be noted. See the Table of Contents to locate the tests listed below.

MONTHLY

Blood Pressure (Heart and Circulation Tests)
Breast Self-Examination (Miscellaneous Tests)
Dental Plaque Disclosure (Miscellaneous Tests)
Pulmonary Function Measurements—Forced Vital Capacity (Breath and Lung Tests)
Skin Observations (Miscellaneous Tests)
Skin Saltiness (Breath and Lung Tests)
Testicle Observations (Genitourinary System Tests)
Urine Tests—using an N-Multistix or Chemstrip 8 dipstick. These screening tests will provide a check on whether urine contains **bilirubin, blood, glucose, ketones, nitrite, protein** and **urobilinogen** as well as its **pH**. Although it is not necessary to evaluate some of the tests included in these dipsticks on a monthly basis, the cost-effectiveness factor makes it worthwhile to use them all.
Weight Observations—Weight alone (Miscellaneous Tests)

QUARTERLY (Every Three Months)

Hearing Function—Voice and Whisper or Ticking Watch (Ear Observations and Hearing Tests)

Hemoglobin (Blood Tests)
Mouth and Throat Observations (Gastrointestinal System Tests)
Visual Acuity (Eye and Vision Tests)
Visual Field (Eye and Vision Tests)

SEMIANNUALLY (Every Six Months)

Dizziness and Ataxia—Finger-to-Nose, Romberg (Brain and Nervous System Tests)
Feces Observations—Occult Blood (Gastrointestinal Systems Tests)
Prostate Observations (Genitourinary System Tests)
Pupillary Reflex (Eye and Vision Tests)
Reflex Testing—Knee-Jerks, Wrist (Brain and Nervous System Tests)

ANNUALLY (Once a Year)

Cold Pressor (Heart and Circulation Tests)
Glucose—Glucose Tolerance Test (Blood tests)
Hair Observations and Mineral Analysis—Anagen-Telogen (Miscellaneous Tests)
Hearing Function—Rinne, Weber (Ear Observations and Hearing Tests)
Pulse Measurements—Two-Step (Exercise) (Heart and Circulation Tests)
Sensory Testing—Graphesthesia (Brain and Nervous System Tests)
Smell Function (Brain and Nervous System Tests)
String Test (Gastrointestinal System Tests)
Urea Nitrogen (Blood Tests)

SPECIAL CIRCUMSTANCES

Before taking any prescription drug and monthly for six months after taking it; monthly if taking drugs regularly:
Capillary Fragility (Heart and Circulation Tests)
Dizziness and Ataxia—Romberg (Brain and Nervous System Tests)
Feces Observations—Occult Blood (Gastrointestinal System Tests)
Hemoglobin (Blood Tests)
Pulse Measurements—Rhythm and Character (Heart and Circulation Tests)
Pupillary Reflex (Eye and Vision Tests)
Urine Tests—using an N-Multistix or Chemstrip 8 dipstick (see tests listed under "Monthly")

Before and monthly for six months after taking drugs known or suspected to affect hearing:

Hearing Function—Audiometer (if possible), Rinne, Ticking Watch, Voice and Whisper, Weber (Ear Observations and Hearing Tests)

Before (and one month after) a woman of childbearing age takes any medicine known or suspected to affect a fetus or before undergoing any X-ray examination:

Breast Self-Examination (Miscellaneous Tests)
Pregnancy (Urine Tests)
Protein (Urine Tests)

On a newborn once a week for the first six weeks of life:

Phenylketonuria Screening (Urine Tests)

APPENDIX II
Disease-Related Index

Most people tend to associate their medical problems with a body organ or some system-related disease. Breathing difficulties are usually attributed to the lungs, but the cause could just as well be secondary to heart and kidney disease. Problems affecting metabolism are first thought to come from the hormone system, or specifically from one of its endocrine glands such as the adrenals, pancreas or thyroid. Discomfort during urination first calls to mind the possibility of kidney and urinary tract disease; sexually transmitted diseases are most likely to be an unwanted afterthought. There are times, however, when a disease is suspected but not to such a degree that professional confirmation is sought, albeit it should be. The following index lists common diseases and indicates home medical tests that can help confirm one's suspicions; unfortunately, medical tests can also belie the presence of a disease, so the test results should be more a matter of prompting one to seek, rather than to avoid, professional medical care. See Table of Contents to locate the tests listed below.

ADRENAL DISEASE

Blood Pressure (Heart and Circulation Tests)
Glucose (Blood Tests)
Protein (Urine Tests)
Specific Gravity (Urine Tests)
Vitamin C Body Level (Miscellaneous Tests)
Weight Observations (Miscellaneous Tests)

ALLERGY

Allergy Patch Testing and Elimination Diet (Miscellaneous Tests)
Body Temperature (Miscellaneous Tests)
Edema (Miscellaneous Tests)
Milk Products (Lactose) Intolerance (Gastrointestinal System Tests)
Pulmonary Function Measurements—Forced Vital Capacity, Match Test (Breath and Lung Tests)

Sinus Transillumination (Miscellaneous Tests)
Skin Infestation—Flea Bites, Pediculosis, Scabies (Miscellaneous Tests)
Skin Observations (Miscellaneous Tests)
Skin Saltiness (Breath and Lung Tests)
Smell Function (Brain and Nervous System Tests)

ANEMIA

Alcoholism (Brain and Nervous System Tests)
Bilirubin (Urine Tests)
Bleeding and Clotting Time (Blood Tests)
Blood (Urine Tests)
Capillary Fragility (Heart and Condition Tests)
Carbon Monoxide (Breath and Lung Tests)
Feces Observations—including Occult Blood and Parasites (Gastrointestinal System Tests)
Hemoglobin (Blood Tests)
Sickle-Cell (Blood Tests)
Skin Observations (Miscellaneous Tests)
String Test (Gastrointestinal System Tests)
Weight Observations (Miscellaneous Tests)

BONE DISEASE

Body Temperature (Miscellaneous Tests)
Hearing Function—Tuning Fork (Ear Observations and Hearing Tests)
Prostate Observations (Genitourinary System Tests)
Protein (Urine Tests)
Rheumatoid Factor (Blood Tests)
Urea Nitrogen (Blood Tests)
Weight Observations (Miscellaneous Test)

BRAIN DISEASE

Alcoholism (Brain and Nervous System Tests)
Blood Pressure (Heart and Circulation Tests)
Body Temperature (Miscellaneous Tests)
Dizziness and Ataxia (Brain and Nervous System Tests)
Glucose (Blood Tests)
Glucose (Urine Tests)
Hearing Function—Weber (Ear Observations and Hearing Tests)
Mental Ability and Personality Testing (Brain and Nervous System Tests)
Phenylketonuria Screening (Urine Tests)

Protein (Urine Tests)
Reflex Testing (Brain and Nervous System Tests)
Sensory Testing (Brain and Nervous System Tests)
Smell Function (Brain and Nervous System Tests)
Taste Function (Brain and Nervous System Tests)
Urea Nitrogen (Blood Tests)
Visual Acuity (Eye and Vision Tests)
Visual Field (Eye and Vision Tests)

CANCER

Blood (Urine Tests)
Breast Self-Examination (Miscellaneous Tests)
Dizziness and Ataxia (Brain and Nervous System Tests)
Feces Observations—Occult Blood (Gastrointestinal System Tests)
Hemoglobin (Blood Tests)
Mouth and Throat Examination (Gastrointestinal System Tests)
Prostate Observations (Genitourinary System Tests)
Protein (Urine Tests)
Pulmonary Function Measurements—Forced Vital Capacity (Breath and Lung Tests)
Skin Observations (Miscellaneous Tests)
Testicle Observations (Genitourinary System Tests)
Urine Flow Rate (Urine Tests)
Vitamin C Body Level (Miscellaneous Tests)
Weight Observations (Miscellaneous Tests)

DENTAL DISEASE

Breath Odor and Sputum (Breath and Lung Tests)
Dental Plaque Disclosure (Miscellaneous Tests)
Hemoglobin (Blood Tests)
Mouth and Throat Examination (Gastrointestinal System Tests)
Sinus Transillumination (Miscellaneous Tests)

DIABETES

Blood Pressure (Heart and Circulation Tests)
Glucose (Blood Tests)
Glucose (Urine Tests)
Ketones (Urine Tests)
Odor (Urine Tests)
Reflex Testing (Brain and Nervous System Tests)
Sensory Testing (Brain and Nervous System Tests)

Skin Observations (Miscellaneous Tests)
Specific Gravity (Urine Tests)
Visual Acuity (Eye and Vision Tests)
Vitamin C (Urine Tests)
Volume (Urine Tests)
Weight Observations (Miscellaneous Tests)

EAR DISEASE

Allergy Patch Testing and Elimination Diet (Miscellaneous Tests)
Dizziness and Ataxia (Brain and Nervous System Tests)
Ear Observations and Hearing Tests

EYE DISEASE

Blood Pressure (Heart and Circulation Tests)
Brain and Nervous System Tests
Cold Face Reflex (Brain and Nervous System Tests)
Edema (Miscellaneous Tests)
Eye and Vision Tests
Glucose (Blood Tests)
Glucose (Urine Tests)
Sinus Transillumination (Miscellaneous Tests)

GASTROINTESTINAL DISEASE

Alcoholism (Brain and Nervous System Tests)
Allergy Patch Testing and Elimination Diet (Miscellaneous Tests)
Blood Pressure (Heart and Circulation Tests)
Gastrointestinal System Tests
Hemoglobin (Blood Tests)
Skin Observations (Miscellaneous Tests)
Skin Saltiness (Breath and Lung Tests)
Smell Function (Brain and Nervous System Tests)
Taste Function (Brain and Nervous System Tests)
Weight Observations (Miscellaneous Tests)

HEART AND CIRCULATORY DISEASE

Alcoholism (Brain and Nervous System Tests)
Carbon Monoxide (Breath and Lung Tests)
Edema (Miscellaneous Tests)
Glucose (Blood Tests)
Glucose (Urine Tests)

Heart and Circulation Tests
Hemoglobin (Blood Tests)
Protein (Urine Tests)
Pulmonary Function Measurements—Forced Vital Capacity (Breath and Lung Tests)
Salt Measurements (Miscellaneous Tests)
Skin Observations (Miscellaneous Tests)
Streptozyme (Blood Tests)
Urea Nitrogen (Blood Tests)
Weight Observations (Miscellaneous Tests)

INFECTIONS

Allergy Patch Testing and Elimination Diet (Miscellaneous Tests)
Body Temperature (Miscellaneous Tests)
Breath Odor and Sputum (Breath and Lung Tests)
Color (Urine Tests)
Dental Plaque Disclosure (Miscellaneous Tests)
Dizziness and Ataxia (Brain and Nervous System Tests)
Ear Canal and Eardrum Observations (Ear Observations and Hearing Tests)
Edema (Miscellaneous Tests)
Feces Observations (Gastrointestinal System Tests)
Gonorrhea (Genitourinary System Tests)
Leukocyte (Blood Tests)
Mononucleosis (Blood Tests)
Mouth and Throat Examination (Gastrointestinal System Tests)
Murphy's Sign (Genitourinary System Tests)
Nitrite (Urine Tests)
Prostate Observations (Genitourinary System Tests)
Protein (Urine Tests)
Pulmonary Function Measurements—Forced Vital Capacity (Breath and Lung Tests)
Pupillary Reflex (Eye and Vision Tests)
Sinus Transillumination (Miscellaneous Tests)
Skin Infestation—Flea Bites, Pediculosis, Scabies (Miscellaneous Tests)
Skin Observations (Miscellaneous Tests)
Streptozyme (Blood Tests)
Two/Three-Glass (Urine Tests)

KIDNEY AND URINARY TRACT DISEASE

Blood Pressure (Heart and Circulation Tests)
Body Temperature (Miscellaneous Tests)
Dizziness and Ataxia (Brain and Nervous System Tests)
Edema (Miscellaneous Tests)

Gonorrhea (Genitourinary System Tests)
Hemoglobin (Blood Tests)
Murphy's Sign (Genitourinary System Tests)
Prostate Observations (Genitourinary System Tests)
Pulmonary Function Measurements—Forced Vital Capacity (Breath and Lung Tests)
Salt Measurements (Miscellaneous Tests)
Urea Nitrogen (Blood Tests)
Urine Tests
Weight Observations (Miscellaneous Tests)

LIVER AND GALLBLADDER DISEASE

Alcoholism (Brain and Nervous System Tests)
Bilirubin (Urine Tests)
Body Temperature (Miscellaneous Tests)
Color (Urine Tests)
Edema (Miscellaneous Tests)
Feces Observations—Color (Gastrointestinal System Tests)
Hemoglobin (Blood Tests)
Mental Ability and Personality Testing—Cognitive Capacity Screening, Number Connection (Brain and Nervous System Tests)
Mononucleosis (Blood Tests)
Protein (Urine Tests)
Skin Observations (Miscellaneous Tests)
Urobilinogen (Urine Tests)

LUNG DISEASE

Allergy Patch Testing and Elimination Diet (Miscellaneous Tests)
Apnea Monitoring (Miscellaneous Tests)
Blood Pressure (Heart and Circulation Tests)
Body Temperature (Miscellaneous Tests)
Breath and Lung Tests
Edema (Miscellaneous Tests)
pH (Urine Tests)
Smell Function (Brain and Nervous System Tests)

MENTAL DISEASE

Alcoholism (Brain and Nervous System Tests)
Allergy Patch Testing and Elimination Diet (Miscellaneous Tests)
Breath Alcohol (Breath and Lung Tests)
Carbon Monoxide (Breath and Lung Tests)

Drug Identification (Miscellaneous Tests)
Glucose (Blood Tests)
Glucose (Urine Tests)
Mental Ability and Personality Testing—Beck Depression Inventory, Cognitive Capacity Screening, Number Connection (Brain and Nervous System Tests)
Mononucleosis (Blood Tests)
Phenylketonuria Screening (Urine Tests)
Smell Function (Brain and Nervous System Tests)
Specific Gravity (Urine Tests)
Taste Function (Brain and Nervous System Tests)
Urea Nitrogen (Blood Tests)

NUTRITIONAL DISEASE

Alcoholism (Brain and Nervous System Tests)
Allergy Patch Testing and Elimination Diet (Miscellaneous Tests)
Breath Odor and Sputum (Breath and Lung Tests)
Capillary Fragility (Heart and Circulation Tests)
Edema (Miscellaneous Tests)
Gastrointestinal System Tests
Glucose (Blood Tests)
Glucose (Urine Tests)
Hemoglobin (Blood Tests)
Ketones (Urine Tests)
Protein (Urine Tests)
Skin Saltiness (Breath and Lung Tests)
Smell Function (Brain and Nervous System Tests)
Taste Function (Brain and Nervous System Tests)
Urea Nitrogen (Blood Tests)
Vitamin C (Urine Tests)
Vitamin C Body Level (Miscellaneous Tests)
Weight Observations (Miscellaneous Tests)

PANCREAS DISEASE

Alcoholism (Brain and Nervous System Tests)
Blood Pressure (Heart and Circulation Tests)
Body Temperature (Miscellaneous Tests)
Feces Observations—Occult Blood (Gastrointestinal System Tests)
Glucose (Blood Tests)
Glucose (Urine Tests)
Protein (Urine Tests)

Skin Saltiness (Breath and Lung Tests)
Weight Observations (Miscellaneous Tests)

PITUITARY DISEASE

Body Temperature (Miscellaneous Tests)
Edema (Miscellaneous Tests)
Glucose (Blood Tests)
Glucose (Urine Tests)
Pupillary Reflex (Eye and Vision Tests)
Smell Function (Brain and Nervous System Tests)
Specific Gravity (Urine Tests)
Visual Acuity (Eye and Vision Tests)
Visual Field (Eye and Vision Tests)
Volume (Urine Tests)
Weight Observations (Miscellaneous Tests)

SEXUALLY RELATED PROBLEMS AND CONDITIONS

Blood (Urine Tests)
Body Temperature (Miscellaneous Tests)
Dizziness and Ataxia (Brain and Nervous System Tests)
Feces Observation—Parasites (Gastrointestinal System Tests)
Gonorrhea (Genitourinary System Tests)
Leukocyte (Urine Tests)
Mental Ability and Personality Testing—Beck Depression Inventory (Brain and Nervous System Tests)
Mononucleosis (Blood Tests)
Mouth and Throat Examination (Gastrointestinal System Tests)
Murphy's Sign (Genitourinary System Tests)
Nitrite (Urine Tests)
Nocturnal Penile Tumescence Screening (Genitourinary System Tests)
Pregnancy (Urine Tests)
Prostate Observations (Genitourinary System Tests)
Pupillary Reflex (Eye and Vision Tests)
Reflex Testing (Brain and Nervous System Tests)
Sensory Testing (Brain and Nervous System Tests)
Skin Infestation—Flea Bites, Pediculosis, Scabies (Miscellaneous Tests)
Skin Observations (Miscellaneous Tests)
Turbidity (Urine Tests)
Two/Three-Glass Test (Urine Tests)
Urine Flow Rate (Urine Tests)

SKIN DISEASE

Allergy Patch Testing and Elimination Diet (Miscellaneous Tests)
Bleeding and Clotting Time (Blood Tests)
Body Temperature (Miscellaneous Tests)
Capillary Fragility (Heart and Circulation Tests)
Color (Urine Tests)
Edema (Miscellaneous Tests)
Feces Observations—Parasites (Gastrointestinal System Tests)
Hair Observations and Mineral Analysis—Anagen-Telogen (Miscellaneous Tests)
Mononucleosis (Blood Tests)
Phenylketonuria Screening (Urine Tests)
Sensory Testing (Brain and Nervous System Tests)
Skin Infestation—Flea Bites, Pediculosis, Scabies (Miscellaneous Tests)
Skin Observations (Miscellaneous Tests)
Skin Saltiness (Breath and Lung Tests)
Streptozyme (Blood Tests)

THYROID DISEASE

Blood Pressure (Heart and Circulation Tests)
Edema (Miscellaneous Tests)
Glucose (Blood Tests)
Glucose (Urine Tests)
Pulmonary Function Measurements—Forced Vital Capacity (Breath and Lung Tests)
Pulse Measurements (Heart and Circulation Tests)
Reflex Testing—Ankle (Brain and Nervous System Tests)
Weight Observations (Miscellaneous Tests)

APPENDIX III
Manufacturer Sources of
Equipment and Supplies

In most instances test equipment and supplies can be obtained through pharmacies, physician and hospital equipment and supply stores, scientific apparatus and instrument stores, and some catalog mail order companies. In the event of difficulty in locating supplies, contact the manufacturer, listed below, directly.

APNEA MONITORS

Abbey Medical Catalog Sales
13782 Crenshaw Blvd.
Gardena, Calif. 90249
(Apnea/Respiration Monitor)

Electronic Monitors, Inc.
P.O. Box 1087
Euless, Texas 76039
(The RE 134 Apnea Monitor)

BLOOD DIPSTICKS (See Dipsticks)

BLOOD GLUCOSE METERS

Ames Division,. Miles Laboratories
Inc.
Elkhart, Ind. 46515
(Glucometer)

LifeScan, Inc.
P.O. Box 1118
Mountain View, Calif. 94042
(Glucoscan)

BLOOD LANCETS, DISPOSABLE

Monoject Division
Sherwood Medical
Brunswick Company
St. Louis, Mo. 63103
(Monolets)

Bio-Dynamics
9115 Hague Rd.
Indianapolis, Ind. 46250
(Autoclix)

BLOOD PRESSURE (See sphygmomanometer)

BLOOD PRICKING DEVICES (Automatic)

Bio-Dynamics
9115 Hague Rd.
Indianapolis, Ind. 46250
(Autoclix)

LifeScan, Inc.
P.O. Box 1118
Mountain View, Calif. 94042
(Penlet)

Ulster Scientific Inc.
P.O. Box 902
Highland, N.Y. 12528
(Autolet)

BODY TEMPERATURE

Trademark Sales Corp.
11501 Concord Village Ave.
St. Louis, Mo. 63128
(Stat-Temp Plastic Fever Detector)

BREAST SCREENING

Faberge Incorporated
1345 Avenue of the Americas
New York, N.Y. 10019
(Breast Cancer Screening Indicator)

BREATH ALCOHOL

Edmund Scientific
101 E. Gloucester Pike
Barrington, N.J. 08007
(Breath Tester)

National Draeger Inc.
P.O. Box 120
Pittsburgh, Pa. 15230
(Alco Test)

The Sharper Image
755 Davis St.
San Francisco, Calif. 94111
(AlcoCheck)

Markline
P.O. Box C–5
Belmont, Mass. 02178
(ATC–1; Direct Reading Alcohol Test
   Computer)

BREATH CARBON MONOXIDE

National Draeger Inc.
P.O. Box 120
Pittsburgh, Pa. 15230
(CO Breath Test)

American Gas & Chemical Co.
220 Pegasus Ave.
Northvale, N.J. 07649
(CO Monitors)

CAPILLARY TUBES

Propper Manufacturing Co. Inc.
Long Island City, N.Y. 11101

DENTAL PLAQUE DISCLOSURE

John O. Butler Co.
Chicago, Ill. 60611
(Instant Red-Cote)

Sultan Chemists Inc.
Englewood, N.J. 07631
(Disclosing Solution)

DIPSTICKS FOR BLOOD AND URINE

Ames Division, Miles Laboratories Inc.
Elkhart, Ind. 46515
(Multistix, Labstix, Chek-Stix, etc.)

Bio-Dynamics
9115 Hague Rd.
Indianapolis, Ind. 46250
(Chemstrips)

Eli Lilly & Co.
740 S. Alabama St.
Indianapolis, Ind. 46206
(TES-TAPE)

GLUCOLA SOLUTION

Ames Division, Miles Laboratories Inc.
Elkhart, Ind. 46515

GONORRHEA

Medical Frontier Enterprieses
P.O. Box 254
Bellbrook, Ohio 45303
(VD ALERT)

United States Packaging Corp.
506 Clay St.
La Porte, Ind. 46350
(GONODECTEN)

HEMOGLOBIN

Medical Charts & Specialties Co.
75 Oser Ave.
Hauppauge, N.Y. 11787
(Tallquist Haemoglobin Scale)

HYDROMETER (See Urinometer)

IMPOTENCE (See Nocturnal Penile Tumescence Stamps)

MILK (LACTOSE) INTOLERANCE

SugarLo Company
P.O. Box 111
Pleasantville, N.J. 08232
(LactAid)

MONONUCLEOSIS BLOOD TEST

Organon Diagnostics
West Orange, N.J. 07052
(Monosticon DRI-DOT)

Wampole Laboratories
Half Acre Rd.
Cranbury, N.J. 08512
(MONO-TEST-FTB)

NOCTURNAL PENILE TUMESCENCE STAMPS

Printing Service
The Oregon Health Sciences Univer-
sity
3181 S.W. Sam Jackson Park Rd.
Portland, Ore. 97201
(NPT stamps)

OCCULT BLOOD

Ames Division, Miles Laboratories
P.O. Box 70
Elkhart, Ind. 46515
(Combistix, Hema-chek, Hematest
tablets)

Bio-Dynamics
9115 Hague Rd.
Indianapolis, Ind. 46250
(Chemstrip 3, Chemstrip 5L)

Helena Laboratories
P.O. Box 752
Beaumont, Texas 77704
(ColoScreen)

Smith Kline Diagnostics
P.O. Box 61947
Sunnyvale, Calif. 94086
(Hemoccult II Slide Test)

URINE FLOW RATE (Peakometer)

Kendall Hospital Products
Boston, Mass. 02101

POCKET MICROSCOPE

Cole-Parmer Instrument Co.
7425 North Oak Park Ave.
Chicago, Ill. 60648
(Pocket Magnifier 30-Power, 100-
Power)

Edmund Scientific
101 E. Gloucester Pike
Barrington, N.J. 08007
(Various Pocket/Pen Microscopes)

Panasonic West Inc.
Division of Matsushita Electric Cor-
poration of America
8383 Wilshire Blvd.
Beverly Hills, Calif. 90211
(Panasonic Light Scope 30-Power)

PREGNANCY TESTS

Carter Products
767 Fifth Ave.
New York, N.Y. 10153
(Answer)

Ortho Pharmaceutical Corp.
Route 202
Raritan, N.J. 08869
(Daisy 2)

Warner-Lambert Co.
201 Tabor Rd.
Morris Plains, N.J. 07950
(e.p.t.)

Whitehall Laboratories
685 Third Ave.
New York, N.Y. 10017
(Predictor)

J.B. Williams Co.
767 Fifth Ave.
New York, N.Y. 10153
(ACU-TEST)

PULSE MONITOR

Hammacher Schlemmer
145 East 57th St.
New York, N.Y. 10022
(The Coach)

ISC Special Products
208 Centerville Rd.
Lancaster, Pa. 17603
(Novatec Digital Pulse Rate Monitor)

The Sharper Image
755 Davis St.
San Francisco, Calif. 94111
(Pulse Tach-Wrist Watch Pulse Monitor Combination)

RADIATION DETECTORS AND MONITORS

Dosimeter Corp.
P.O. Box 42377
Cincinnati, Ohio 45242
(Dosimeters, Monitors, Rechargers)

The Sharper Image
755 Davis St.
San Francisco, Calif. 94111
(Personal Geiger Counter)

The 3-M Company
St. Paul, Minn. 55144
(Tan-Timer)

RDX Nuclear
2003 Canyon Dr.
Los Angeles, Calif. 90068
(DX-1 Geiger Counter)
measures beta and gamma

REFLEX HAMMER

American Hospital Supply
1450 Waukegan Rd.
Mcgaw Park, Ill. 60085
(rubber percussion hammer)

RHEUMATOID FACTOR BLOOD TEST

Organon Diagnostics
West Orange, N.J. 07052
(RHEUMANOSTICAN DRI-DOT)

SALT MEASURING METER

Life Power Products Inc.
5316 West Imperial Highway
Los Angeles, Calif. 90045
(Original Salt Meter)

SICKLE-CELL BLOOD TEST

Ortho Pharmaceutical Corp.
Route 202
Raritan, N.J. 08869
(SICKLEDEX)

SINUS TRANSILLUMINATOR

American Optical Corp.
Eggert and Sugar Roads
Buffalo, N.Y. 14215
(Battery Transilluminator)

Welch Allyn Inc.
Jordan Rd.
Skaneateles Falls, N.Y. 13153
(Ear/Nose/Throat Transilluminator)

SKINFOLD CALIPERS

Abbey Medical Catalog Sales
13782 Crenshaw Blvd.
Gardena, Calif. 90249
(The Lange Skinfold Caliper)

Ross Laboratories Division
Abbott Laboratories
Columbus, Ohio 43216
(Nutritional Assessment Kit)

SOUND LEVEL METER

Radio Shack Stores
Tandy Corporation
Fort Worth, Texas 76102
(Realistic Sound Level Meter)

SPHYGMOMANOMETER

The Lumiscope Company Inc.
836 Broadway
New York, N.Y. 10003
(Digital Electronic Blood Pressure
Unit with Built-in Pulse Meter)

Sears Roebuck and Co.
Sears Tower
Chicago, Ill. 60684
(see Home Health Care Catalog)

SPIROMETERS

Armstrong Industries Inc.
P.O. Box 7
Northbrook, Ill. 60062
(Mini-Wright Peak Flow Meter)

Propper Manufacturing Co. Inc.
36–04 Skillman Ave.
Long Island City, N.Y. 11101
(Spirometer)

Vitalograph Ltd.
8347 Quivira Rd.
Lenexa, Kan. 66215
(Pulmonary Monitor with Peak Flow
  Scale)

Kinetics Measurement Corp.
Sterling Lake Rd.
Tuxedo, N.Y. 10987
(Windmill)

Organon Hospital Products
West Orange, N.J. 07052
(Peak Flow Meter)

STREPTOCOCCUS BLOOD TEST

Wampole Laboratories
Half Acre Rd.
Cranbury, N.J. 08512
(STREPTOZYME)

STRING TEST

HEDECO Health Development Corp.
2551 Casey Ave.
Mountain View, Calif. 94043
(Entero-Test)

TUNING FORK

American Hospital Supply
1450 Waukegan Rd.
Mcgaw Park, Ill. 60085

UREA NITROGEN BLOOD TEST

Ames Division, Miles Laboratories Inc.
Elkhart, Inc. 46515
(AZOSTIX)

URINE DIPSTICKS (See Dipsticks)

URINOMETER

E.R. Squibb and Sons Inc.
P.O. Box 4000
Princeton, N.J. 08540

VISION TESTING

Medical Charts and Specialties Co.
75 Oser Ave.
Haupauge, N.Y. 11787
(Snellen Eye Chart, color-blindness
testing plates)